SOMATIC EXERCISES FOR WEIGHT LOSS

A Comprehensive Guide To Transformative Training Technique, Holistic Exercises For Effortless Weight Loss, Stress Reduction And Enhanced Emotional Well-Being

Linda S. Samson

Table Of Contents

CHAPTER 1: INTRODUCTION TO SOMATIC EXERCISE

In a world where the search for health may seem like an elusive quest, with fad diets and hard exercises dominating the talk around weight reduction, there is a revolutionary and often ignored approach: somatic exercise. This book delves into the world of somatic exercise, revealing its promise as a conscious and comprehensive approach to weight control.

Somatic exercise is more than just a physical regimen; it is a journey that explores the complex relationship between the mind and body. Unlike traditional fitness approaches, which are primarily concerned with outward outcomes, somatic exercise challenges us to gaze within, tapping into the wisdom housed within our bodies. It is a strategy that promotes a healthy balance between the body, mind, and spirit, resulting in not just weight reduction but also a holistic feeling of well-being.

To begin this somatic journey, we must first break free from the constraints of conventional weight reduction procedures. Calorie counting and intense exercises often dominate the narrative, resulting in a cycle of transient success followed by unavoidable relapse. Somatic exercise encourages us to reevaluate these misconceptions, providing a paradigm shift that goes beyond the constraints of traditional thinking. It's an encouragement to adopt a sustainable, conscientious, and very individualized approach to weight control.

Somatic exercise is based on a deep awareness of the mind-body relationship. Our nervous system, a complex network of neurons and synapses, regulates not just our movements but also our reactions to stress and emotions. Somatics taps into this link, allowing us to control stress hormones and develop a greater awareness of our bodies. The somatic method focuses on soft motions that feed rather than burden the body. We look at workouts that increase posture, flexibility, and core strength without using force, but rather via focused participation.

The trip includes a dance including multiple somatic movement modalities—Feldenkrais, BodyMind Centering, and Pilates—each presenting a distinct viewpoint on the transformational power of conscious movement. Somatic exercise emphasizes breathing, which is typically disregarded in standard weight control regimes. We explore the complex relationship between breath and weight, learning how aware breathing may control metabolism, decrease stress, and promote emotional balance. Practical breathing exercises become tools for incorporating awareness into our everyday lives, laying the groundwork for long-term weight balance.

Weight control goes beyond physical exercise; it is intertwined with our eating habits. Cultivating attentive eating habits becomes a cornerstone of the somatic approach. This entails breaking away from the cycle of emotional eating, developing habits of aware food choices, and adopting portion management as a kind of self-care. The focus switches to developing a specific somatic exercise regimen. This is not a one-size-fits-all routine, but rather an encouragement to create a practice that suits your lifestyle, tastes, and individual body.

We investigate how to smoothly incorporate somatic exercises into everyday life, guaranteeing a constant and joyful experience with this transforming journey. Recognizing that somatic exercise is not an independent undertaking, we investigate the relationship between somatics and nutrition. Mindful eating choices magnify the influence of somatic activities, resulting in a more comprehensive approach to weight control that feeds both the body and mind.

The road to conscious weight control is not without its hurdles. Throughout this trip, we identify typical challenges and provide techniques for long-term commitment. It acknowledges that meaningful change is more than just fast cures; it is a commitment to a lifetime connection with one's well-being. Somatics invites us to explore the greater advantages it provides for general health. It's an encouragement to embrace sustainable health behaviors that go beyond the scale, resulting in a more meaningful and balanced existence.

In the following pages, we will start on a journey of self-discovery, revealing the wisdom of somatic exercise for weight loss and, more importantly, for a life lived with mindful purpose. This is more than a book; it is an invitation to a transforming experience—one that goes beyond the constraints of conventional weight reduction and introduces a comprehensive and sustainable approach to well-being. Welcome to the revolution, where weight reduction and self-discovery intersect, and each stride forward is a whispered conversation with your own gorgeous body.

1.1 What is Somatic Exercise?

Somatic exercise is a method of movement and body awareness that focuses on engaging the mind and body simultaneously. It entails thoughtful and deliberate movements that enhance posture, flexibility, and general physical function. Somatic exercises often emphasize internal awareness, urging participants to focus on sensations, sentiments, and movement quality. Somatic exercises entail just moving to move. Throughout the workout, you concentrate on your inner experience while moving and expanding your inside awareness.

The term "somatic" derives from the word "soma," which refers to the living organism in its whole, including the intellect. Somatic exercises are intended to address and relieve muscle tension, improve coordination, and foster a stronger feeling of body awareness. Somatics leverages the mind-body link to assist you in surveying your interior self and listening to your body's indications of pain, discomfort, or imbalance. Somatic therapy includes this approach to mental health treatment.

Somatic exercise practitioners often experiment with several modalities such as Feldenkrais, BodyMind Centering, and some aspects of Pilates. These techniques stress gentle movements and the mind-body connection to reeducate the nervous system and enhance general movement patterns. Somatic exercise is not your average gym session. It's a distinct style of movement that emphasizes internal awareness, mind-body connection, and gentle exploration of your body's potential. Here's what makes it stand out:

1. *Focus on Internal Experience*: Unlike conventional fitness, which emphasizes outward objectives such as muscle building or calorie burning, somatic exercise focuses on how you feel inside while exercising. You become more aware of subtle sensations, experiment with varied ranges of motion, and appreciate your body's sophisticated workings.

2. *Gentle and Mindful Movement*: Forget about working yourself to exhaustion. Somatic workouts are frequently slow, meticulous, and emphasize accuracy over intensity. It is about paying attention to your breathing, joint alignment, and muscle engagement.

3. Rewiring the Nervous System: Somatic exercise, which combines soft movements and focused awareness, may help regulate your nervous system and decrease stress. This may result in better posture, less discomfort, and a more relaxed mental state, all of which benefit your overall health.

4. Building Functional Strength: Do not be deceived by the easy motions. Somatic exercise may significantly enhance strength, flexibility, and coordination. You'll develop the functional strength that your body needs for daily tasks, not simply dazzling gym accomplishments.

5. Breaking the Diet Mentality: By building a deep connection to your body's internal signals, somatic exercise may help you transition away from restrictive diets and toward a more intuitive relationship with food. You'll learn to listen to your body's hunger and fullness cues and make deliberate decisions based on your requirements.

6. *Benefits Beyond the Physical*: The profound influence of somatic exercise goes beyond the physical sphere. It may increase self-compassion, enhance body image, and foster a feeling of inner calm. By learning to move with awareness and acceptance, you'll get a new respect for your unique body and its talents.

1.2 Introducing the Transforming Potential of Somatics Exercise for Mindful Weight Control

For decades, the story around weight control has been a dull, repeated mantra of "calories in, calories out," strenuous exercises, and restricted diets. It's a story about frustration, plateaus, and the ongoing battle against your own body. What if there was another way? A manner that goes beyond the physical warfare of the gym and explores the deeper worlds of mind-body connection, intentional movement, and a deep respect for your body's wisdom? This is where the transforming potential of somatic exercise for conscious weight control comes into play.

Somatic exercise does not include pushing oneself to the point of fatigue or copying the artificial motions of fitness equipment. It's about gently rediscovering your body's language, conversing softly with your muscles and neurological system, and practicing movement in sync with your inner rhythms. It's about moving with awareness, purpose, and realizing that genuine sustenance comes from within, not simply from the food on your plate.

Somatic exercise, unlike its typical fitness equivalents, is not concerned with chasing calorie deficits or molding your body into a certain shape. Instead, it fosters a thorough listening practice, transforming you into a conscious observer of your inner world. You learn to detect your body's delicate signals of hunger, fullness, tension, and energy levels. This introspective journey promotes a tremendous shift in which you cease to be at odds with your body and instead become its partner, gently leading it toward health and wellness.

But how does a mindful approach to movement relate to weight management? The explanation lies in the complex relationship between the mind and body. When you perform somatic exercises like Feldenkrais, BodyMind Centering, or mild yogic movements, you are not simply working your muscles; you are also rewiring brain pathways, lowering stress hormones, and promoting a more relaxed emotional state. This, in turn, affects your connection with food, allowing you to break away from emotional eating habits and make mindful decisions based on your body's genuine requirements rather than cravings caused by stress or worry.

Somatic training also helps you avoid the stiff, sometimes painful motions that many gym programs require. By concentrating on soft, methodical movements that value form and awareness over intensity, you may lay the groundwork for functional strength, flexibility, and posture that will benefit your whole body. This newfound connection to your physical self enables you to move with grace and ease, shedding not just pounds but also the restrictive attitudes and negative self-talk that so frequently accompany conventional weight reduction efforts.

Somatic exercise has a transformational force that reaches beyond the physical world, affecting your emotional and mental well-being. Mindful movement promotes self-compassion and body positivity. You learn to applaud any improvement, no matter how tiny, and to accept your body's particular knowledge. This change in attitude leads to a long-term, holistic approach to weight control that prioritizes your total health and well-being above the numbers on the scale.

Of course, the route to conscious weight control with somatic exercise requires commitment and endurance. It's about listening to your body's tiny signs, understanding its language, and developing a strong faith in its intrinsic knowledge. However, the benefits outweigh any number on the scale. You'll get a new respect for your physical shape, a feeling of empowered self-care, and a profound connection to yourself that goes beyond the surface chase of an ideal weight.

So, if you're seeking a weight loss strategy that goes beyond the gym and calorie counting, consider the transformational impact of somatic exercise. Begin your journey with moderate movements inspired by awareness and purpose. Listen to your body, appreciate its knowledge, and move gracefully and effortlessly. You'll be astonished by how much this thoughtful approach can improve your relationship with food, your physical health, and your total sense of self. Remember that mindful weight management isn't about battling your body; it's about working with it to achieve self-discovery, acceptance, and overall well-being. Take the initial step, speak to your muscles, and move with your breath. Your body is prepared to lead you on a transformative path of mindful weight control.

CHAPTER 2: UTILIZING THE MIND-BODY CONNECTION

2.1 Understanding the Neurological System's Impact on Weight Regulation

The battleground of calories and exercise has been the focus of weight control efforts. We diligently count and burn them off, yet the obstinate pounds frequently hang on despite our best efforts. But what if the answer to long-term weight management lay not in our muscles and meals, but in the complicated network of our neurological system? In the complicated dance of human physiology, the nervous system emerges as the orchestrator, exerting significant control over a wide range of body activities, including the complex world of weight management. Let dive into the nerve system's labyrinthine pathways, revealing how they shape our connection with weight and how somatic exercises may be used to promote conscious weight control.

Our nerve system, the quiet director of our internal symphony, plays a subtle but crucial function in weight regulation. It's a complex symphony of nerves, hormones, and neurotransmitters that continuously deliver messages that affect everything from food digestion to fat storage and metabolism. Understanding this complicated dance becomes critical in our pursuit of good weight control. At the heart of our being, the nervous system reigns supreme, serving as the command center for every aspect of our physiological and psychological life. The nervous system, which is made up of the brain and spinal cord, as well as a complicated network of peripheral nerves, is responsible for coordinating reactions to external and internal stimuli.

When it comes to weight control, the nervous system acts like a sophisticated regulator, continually receiving and processing information from the body and its surroundings. Its effect goes beyond the mechanics of movement and sensation, into metabolism, hormone balance, and stress response—a complex web of interrelated systems that define the makeup of our bodies.

2.1.1 The Sympathetic and Parasympathetic Nervous Systems:

Consider two conductors in your nervous system, both competing for control: the sympathetic nervous system and the parasympathetic nervous system. When confronted with stress or danger, our sympathetic system, or fight-or-flight conductor, increases adrenaline levels. It triggers the production of cortisol, a strong hormone that causes the body to store energy and accumulate fat. When stress becomes chronic, cortisol levels stay high, resulting in a metabolic imbalance that may cause weight gain.

The parasympathetic system, or our rest-and-digest conductor, encourages relaxation and healing. It initiates the "feed and breed" response, which promotes digestion, nutritional absorption, and energy expenditure. When the parasympathetic nervous system takes control, our bodies are poised for optimum metabolic activity, which promotes appropriate weight management.

2.1.2 The Orchestra of Hormones: Decoding Chemical Messengers

The neurological system's impact on weight extends beyond cortisol. Neurotransmitters such as leptin and ghrelin play an important role in controlling appetite and satiation. Fat cells produce leptin, which indicates fullness, while the stomach secretes ghrelin, which promotes appetite. Chronic stress upsets this delicate balance, causing leptin resistance and increased ghrelin production, which encourages overeating and weight gain.

2.1.3 Disrupting the Metabolic Symphony:

The contemporary world is a continual symphony of stress, ranging from demanding work to financial concerns. Chronic stress activates the sympathetic nervous system, flooding our bodies with cortisol and upsetting the delicate balance of our metabolic symphony. What are the consequences? Increased visceral fat deposition, particularly in the belly, decreased insulin sensitivity, and impaired glucose metabolism, all contribute to weight gain and obesity-related health concerns.

2.1.4 Restoring Harmony: Tuning the Nervous System for Weight Management.

The good news is that we are not only passive participants in this metabolic symphony. We may learn to adjust our neurological system and maximize its impact on weight management. Here are a few major strategies:

1. *Stress Management:* Chronic stress contributes significantly to weight growth. Prioritize stress-relieving activities such as meditation, yoga, mindfulness, and spending time outside. These activities stimulate the parasympathetic nervous system, which promotes relaxation and metabolic balance.

2. *Sleep Hygiene:* Sleep deprivation impairs hormone homeostasis, resulting in increased cortisol and reduced leptin, which promotes appetite and weight gain. Set regular sleep patterns, create a calming evening ritual, and limit screen time before bed.

3. *Mindful Eating:* When we eat in a hurry or under stress, our nervous system stays in fight-or-flight mode, which impedes digestion and nutritional absorption. Savor your meal, chew properly, and pay attention to hunger and fullness signs.

4. *Exercise for Balance*: While not the only solution, moderate exercise may assist regulate the neurological system. Choose activities that you love, practice mindful movement, and avoid pushing yourself to fatigue. Regular exercise may aid with stress reduction, sleep improvement, and mood enhancement, all of which contribute to good weight control.

2.1.5 Mind-Body Connections and Weight Regulation:

Understanding the nervous system's role in weight management reminds us that our physical health is inextricably linked to our mental and emotional well-being. Addressing stress, prioritizing self-care, and developing a positive body image are essential for long-term weight control.

Navigating the neurological system's maze in our search for weight management is a continuous process, not a fast remedy. It requires self-awareness, a dedication to gentle techniques, and an appreciation for the intricate interaction of our ideas, emotions, and bodily reactions. By learning to listen to our bodies, manage stress, and nurture a holistic approach to well-being, we may start to harmonize the internal symphony, opening the way for a better, happier connection with ourselves and our bodies.

2.1.6 The Vagus Nerve:

Among the extensive network of the autonomic nervous system, the vagus nerve emerges as a vital component in brain-body communication. This cranial nerve, noted for its many connections to organs in the chest and belly, functions as a bidirectional communication conduit. It not only transmits information from the brain to the body, but it also returns impulses from the body to the brain.

The vagus nerve balances the sympathetic and parasympathetic neural systems, controlling the body's rest-and-digest responses. Activation of the vagus nerve promotes relaxation, digestion, and a general sense of calm, in contrast to the sympathetic nervous system's activation caused by stress. Through this delicate balance, the vagus nerve may influence metabolism and, as a result, weight management.

Somatic techniques that focus on relaxation, diaphragmatic breathing, and gentle movements are essential for activating the vagus nerve. Individuals who engage in behaviors that stimulate the parasympathetic nervous system may offset the effects of chronic stress, creating a more conducive environment for weight management.

2.1.7 Somatic Exercises as Nervous System Modulators:

The complex interaction between the neurological system and weight control emphasizes the importance of somatic workouts as powerful modulators of this connection. Somatic exercises, with their focus on attentive movements and conscious awareness, provide a novel approach to negotiating the complexity of the nervous system's impact on weight.

1. Mindful Movement and Stress Reduction: Somatic exercises emphasize gentle, focused movements that engage both the mind and the body in harmony. Individuals may break the cycle of chronic stress by moving with awareness, allowing the nervous system to rest from the pressures of contemporary life.

2. Breathwork as a Nervous System Regulator: Conscious breathing, which is central to many somatic practices, has a direct influence on the autonomic nervous system. Deep, diaphragmatic breathing activates the vagus nerve, causing a transition to the parasympathetic state. This not only relieves stress but also helps to create a more favorable hormonal environment for weight control.

3. *Enhancing Body Awareness:* Somatic activities provide a greater feeling of bodily awareness. Individuals may identify probable causes of stress by tuning into internal sensations and detecting regions of tension or discomfort, and then treat them via deliberate movement and relaxation.

4. *The Role of Proprioception:* Proprioception is an important aspect of somatic exercises because it allows the body to detect its position and movement. Individuals may enhance coordination, balance, and movement patterns by honing their proprioceptive awareness, all of which affect the nervous system's reaction to stress and its effect on weight.

5. *Vagal Tone Enhancement*: Somatic activities that target the stimulation of the vagus nerve helps to increase vagal tone. This, in turn, promotes nervous system equilibrium and creates an atmosphere favorable to conscious weight control.

2.1.8 The Somatic Journey Toward Balance:

Starting a somatic journey for weight loss requires understanding the interwoven web of the nerve system's effect. It is an invitation to investigate movement, breath, and mindfulness as methods for regulating the complex relationship between stress, hormones, and weight.

Individuals who participate in somatic exercises progressively reorganize the neurological networks that control their reactions to stress. The focus on gentle movements, intentional breathwork, and increased bodily awareness serves as a means of recalibrating the nervous system's default mode, directing it away from chronic stress and toward homeostasis. In the arena of somatic exercise, the nervous system converts from a potential opponent, prolonging stress-induced weight difficulties, to an ally in the quest for conscious weight control. Individuals may develop an environment for holistic well-being by traversing the complicated pathways of the neurological system with purpose and attention.

2.2 Utilizing Stress Modulation as a Strategy for Mindful Weight Management

In the fast-paced tapestry of contemporary life, stress has become a ubiquitous force, influencing not just our everyday experiences but also having a significant influence on our bodies. Let investigates the complex link between stress and weight, revealing the physiological processes at work. Furthermore, it investigates how stress control, when tackled thoughtfully via somatic exercises, might emerge as an effective strategy for obtaining and maintaining a healthy weight.

For those of us struggling with our weight, the gym may seem like a war, with the calorie counter as a weapon and our bodies as the enemy. We push, count, and deny, yet the elusive goal of conscious weight management remains out of grasp. But what if the secret to achieving a healthy body weight isn't only counting calories and doing crunches, but also quieting the internal battle cry of stress?

Stress, the ubiquitous bogeyman of the contemporary world, has a profound, although frequently underestimated, impact on our weight. It affects more than just our frazzled nerves and tightening belts; it orchestrates a nuanced ballet inside our neural system, a dance that has the potential to tilt the scales the wrong way.

2.2.1 The Stress and Weight Connection:

Stress, in its different manifestations, initiates a series of physiological reactions that prepare the body for urgent action—the well-known "fight or flight" response. While this acute stress reaction is adaptive in the face of imminent dangers, chronic stress, which is common in our contemporary lives, may cause a variety of health problems, including weight concerns.

When stress becomes chronic, the body reacts by secreting cortisol, the principal stress hormone. Elevated cortisol levels promote fat accumulation, especially visceral fat—fat that collects around organs in the abdomen. This occurrence has been related to an increased risk of metabolic diseases, cardiovascular disease, and other health problems.

Chronic stress often alters eating habits, in addition to having a direct impact on fat accumulation. For many people, stress triggers emotional eating, which is defined by the ingestion of high-calorie, frequently sweet, or fatty meals, as a coping technique. The interaction of stress, cortisol, and eating patterns forms a complicated web that may lead to weight gain and impede weight loss attempts.

2.2.2 Somatic Approach to Stress Regulation:
Among the problems faced by chronic stress, the somatic method emerges as a beacon of hope—a means to consciously control stress and foster a state of homeostasis that promotes mindful weight management. Somatic activities, which focus on deliberate movements, breath awareness, and increased body sense, become useful tools for managing the complex link between stress and weight.

1. *Gentle Movements for Stress Relief:* Somatic exercises focus on gentle, focused movements that relieve muscle tension and promote relaxation. Individuals who engage in these motions may break the cycle of chronic stress, promoting a more harmonious interaction between body and mind.

2. *Breathwork for Stress Reduction:* Conscious breathing, which is a key component of many somatic practices, is an effective stress-reduction strategy. Deep, diaphragmatic breathing triggers the parasympathetic nerve system, or "rest and digest" response, which counteracts the physiological consequences of prolonged stress. When people include breathwork into their everyday routines, they build a bridge to a calmer, more balanced state that aids in weight management.

3. *Mindful Awareness and Stress Response:* Somatic exercises improve physical awareness, enabling people to detect early signals of stress in their bodies. This increased awareness serves as a trigger for proactive stress management, allowing people to react before stress rises and adversely affects eating habits or hormonal balance.

4. *Neural Repatterning:* Chronic stress may cause neural patterns that strengthen the stress response. Somatic activities provide a unique chance for neural repatterning. Individuals may rewire their neural systems by participating in deliberate relaxation-promoting movements and activities, moving away from typical stress reactions and toward more adaptive, calm states.

5. *Embracing the Relaxation Response:* Somatic activities help to activate the relaxation response, which is a physiological condition characterized by a slower heart rate, lower blood pressure, and a sensation of peace. Individuals who frequently engage in relaxation-inducing methods build a stress-resilient foundation that promotes mindful weight management.

2.2.3 Mindful Eating and Emotion Regulation:

Beyond the physiological impacts of stress, somatic exercises help with conscious weight management by addressing the emotional aspects of eating choices. Many people who are attempting to control their weight struggle with emotional eating, which is often driven by stress. Somatic techniques, with their emphasis on awareness and emotional control, are useful aids in this area of weight management.

1. *Cultivating Mindful Eating Habits:* Somatic exercises promote mindful eating. Individuals may break away from the autopilot of emotional eating by increasing their awareness of taste, texture, and the process of eating itself, allowing them to make more intentional, wholesome meal choices.

*2. **Breaking the Cycle of Emotional Eating:*** Somatic exercises provide people with non-food-based stress coping techniques. Individuals who include relaxation methods and mindful exercise in their everyday routines might stop the pattern of utilizing food as a key strategy of emotional control.

*3. **Emotional Awareness and Body Connection:*** Somatic techniques strengthen the link between emotions and physical sensations. Individuals might get insight into the core reasons for emotional eating by understanding their physical manifestations inside the body. This increased awareness catalyzes transformation, helping people to address underlying emotional causes more effectively.

2.2.4 Somatic Exercises for Daily Stress Management:

As people traverse the complexity of stress and weight control via somatic exercises, incorporating these practices into everyday life becomes more important. This section delves into practical, common somatic activities that people may do to relieve stress and assist their weight control objectives.

1. *Body Scan Meditation:* This simple yet effective technique includes bringing concentrated attention to various regions of the body, gradually relieving tension and fostering relaxation. This mindfulness approach enables people to develop an awareness of their physical sensations while disconnecting from stress.

2. *Diaphragmatic Breathing:* A fundamental breathwork method in somatic practices, diaphragmatic breathing triggers the relaxation response. Individuals may soothe their nervous systems by breathing deeply into the diaphragm and thoroughly exhaling, lowering cortisol levels and encouraging emotional equilibrium.

3. *Mindful Walking:* This ordinary activity is transformed into a mindful practice by paying attention to each step, the feelings in the feet, and the rhythm of the breath. This simple yet powerful somatic practice increases grounding, decreases tension, and provides an opportunity for emotional control.

4. *Progressive Muscle Relaxation (PMR)*: Somatics exercise that improves total relaxation by gradually tensing and then releasing various muscle groups. Individuals relieve physical stress by releasing muscular tension, which also creates a route to mental well-being.

5. *Somatic Movement Sequences:* Gentle, deliberate movement sequences serve to relieve accumulated muscle tension and promote the flow of energy throughout the body. Somatic movement becomes a dynamic manifestation of stress control, giving people a toolset for staying balanced in the face of everyday pressures.

2.2.5 The Holistic Effect of Somatic Stress Regulation:

Individuals who begin on a somatic journey for stress management and weight reduction often find a comprehensive change that goes beyond the physical features of their bodies. Somatic techniques open the door to a deeper awareness of oneself, encouraging resilience, self-compassion, and a feeling of strength in the face of life's adversities.

1. *Resilience to Life's Challenges:* Somatic activities promote resilience by training people to react to challenges with awareness and purpose. This resilience protects against the harmful effects of prolonged stress on weight and general well-being.

2. *Self-Compassion:* Mindful stress control via somatic exercises promotes a loving attitude toward one's challenges. Instead of perceiving stress as a failure, people learn to accept their difficulties with compassion, resulting in a supportive internal environment that improves emotional well-being.

3. *Empowerment in Self-Care:* Somatic practices enable people to take an active part in their self-care. Individuals who include stress-reduction activities in their daily routines recover agency over their well-being, promoting a feeling of control and mastery in the face of life's challenges.

The incorporation of somatic exercises into stress management becomes an effective method for attaining and sustaining conscious weight control.

Individuals may approach weight management holistically by realizing the connection between stress, hormones, and emotional eating, which includes deliberate exercise, breath awareness, and increased physical sensing.

Somatic exercises not only help you navigate the complex link between stress and weight, but they also encourage a transformational journey to a more conscious and balanced existence. Individuals who embrace the somatic approach to stress management start on a lifetime companionate relationship with their bodies, transcending the constraints of traditional weight control approaches and inviting them into a world of self-discovery, resilience, and empowered well-being.

CHAPTER 3: RETHINKING WEIGHT LOSS MYTHS

3.1 Breaking Away from Traditional Calorie Formulae

The conventional approach to weight control has long been governed by a simple equation: calories in vs calories out. This reductionist approach, although seeming rational, oversimplifies the body's complicated connection with food. This chapter examines the limits of standard calorie formulae and calls for a somatic approach—a nuanced and thoughtful method that moves beyond the numerical concentration on calories to support a long-term journey toward weight control and general well-being.

3.1.1 The Calorie Conundrum:

The conventional knowledge regarding weight control centers on the idea that weight is governed by the balance between calories ingested and calories expended. According to this paradigm, weight gain happens when calories taken exceed calories burnt; weight decrease occurs when calories burned exceed calories consumed. While this equation offers a fundamental foundation, it oversimplifies the complex interactions between the body, metabolism, and the quality of calories eaten.

3.1.2 The Drawbacks of Caloric Reductionism:

The calorie calculation often succumbs to reductionist thinking, seeing the body as a simple mathematical mechanism. However, the human body is a dynamic and adaptable creature, with many elements affecting its reaction to food that go beyond caloric quantity.

1. Nutrient Quality: Not all calories are created equally. Traditional calorie formulae overlook the significance of dietary quality. Consuming nutrient-dense meals versus empty-calorie, processed foods may have quite different effects on general health and weight control.

2. Metabolic Variability: Every person's metabolism is unique, and impacted by genetics, hormone balance, and general health. Traditional calorie formulae fail to account for the variation in metabolic rates across individuals.

3. Hormonal Management: The hormonal response to eating is critical in weight management. For example, the body reacts differently to a high-sugar meal than it does to a balanced, nutrient-dense one. Traditional calorie formulae often neglect these hormonal differences.

4. *Psychological Factors:* Stress, mood, and eating habits may all have a big influence on food choices and metabolism. Traditional calorie formulae ignore the complex link between mental health and weight.

3.1.3 The Somatic Paradigm:

Somatic methods for weight control differ from a strict emphasis on calorie arithmetic. Instead, they promote a comprehensive awareness of the body-mind relationship, stressing the qualitative elements of food, mindful eating, and the effects of stress on metabolism. This paradigm shift offers a more complete framework for those seeking long-term and conscious weight management.

3.1.4 Mindful Eating:

The somatic method is based on mindful eating, which goes beyond mechanical calorie monitoring to foster awareness, appreciation, and attunement to the body's signals and the sensory experience of eating.

1. *Cultivating Presence:* Mindful eating encourages people to be completely present during meals, relishing every mouthful and paying attention to hunger and satiety signals. This technique promotes a stronger connection with the eating experience, increasing enjoyment while decreasing the probability of overeating.

2. *Emotional Resonance:* Somatic techniques acknowledge the emotional impact of eating choices. Mindful eating encourages people to investigate the emotional triggers that drive eating patterns, therefore addressing the underlying reasons for overeating or bad food choices.

3. *Breaking Free from Restriction:* Traditional calorie-focused diets frequently encourage restrictive behaviors, categorizing foods as "good" or "bad." Somatic approaches, on the other hand, promote a balanced and intuitive approach to eating, recognizing that all foods can play a role in a healthy, varied diet.

3.1.5 Somatic Impact on Metabolism:

Somatic practices have an impact on metabolic processes that are affected by stress, emotions, and general well-being, in addition to the act of eating.

1. Stress Reduction: Chronic stress causes the production of cortisol, a hormone associated with increased belly fat accumulation. Somatic techniques, which emphasize stress reduction via conscious movement and breathwork, help to create a more balanced hormonal environment that promotes weight control.

2. Enhancing Metabolic Flexibility: Somatic workouts increase metabolic flexibility, which is the body's dynamic capacity to effectively transition between carbs and lipids for energy. This adaptation is critical for maintaining energy balance and avoiding the accumulation of excess calories as fat.

3. *Hormonal Harmony:* Somatic techniques understand the complex interplay of hormones in weight control. Individuals may nurture hormonal balance via mindful activities, which makes the body more open to long-term weight management.

3.1.6 The Role of Nutrient-Dense Eating:

Rather than focusing on calorie counts, somatic techniques promote the consumption of nutrient-dense whole meals. This transition from quantitative to qualitative considerations stresses food's nutritional worth and influence on overall health and well-being.

1. *Micronutrient Richness:* Somatic methods promote the intake of foods high in vitamins, minerals, and antioxidants, which have important roles in metabolism, cellular function, and general health.

2. *Satisfying the Body's Needs:* By emphasizing nutrient-dense foods, people are better able to satisfy their body's nutritional requirements. This not only promotes healthy performance but also lessens cravings for less nutrient-dense meals.

3. *Long-Term Nutrition:* Traditional calorie-focused diets often provide short-term weight reduction followed by rebound effects. Somatic methods, based on nutrient-dense eating, promote long-term sustenance and sustainability, promoting a positive connection with food.

3.1.7 Implementing Somatic Practices for Sustainable Weight Management:

Practical ideas and information on how to incorporate somatic practices into their everyday life for long-term weight control.

I. Somatic Movement Routine:

1. Morning Mindful Movement: Begin each day with simple somatic movements. Stretch, breathe, and become aware of the feelings in your body. This creates a pleasant tone for the day and promotes attentive activity.

2. Stress-Busting Breaks: Incorporate brief somatic exercises into your daily routine to reduce stress. Whether it's a fast body scan, a short breathing exercise, or moderate stretches, these pauses help reset your nervous system and lessen the physiological effects of stress.

3. *Mindful Eating Practices:* Set a quiet and focused eating atmosphere. Chew your meal gently and relish every mouthful. Pay attention to hunger and fullness cues, and let your body's natural signals guide your eating.

II. Breathing Exercises for Stress Reduction:

1. *Diaphragmatic Breathing:* Practice diaphragmatic breathing regularly. Sit comfortably, with one hand on your chest and the other on your abdomen. Inhale deeply through your nostrils, allowing your stomach to rise, and exhale gradually through your mouth. This practice calms the nervous system and promotes a state of relaxation.

2. *Box Breathing:* Inhale for four counts, hold for four counts, exhale for four counts, then pause for four more. Repeat this box breathing pattern for a few minutes to relax and decrease tension.

3. Breath Awareness Meditation: Set out a few minutes each day to practice breath awareness meditation. Concentrate your focus on the natural rhythm of your breathing, watching without judgment. This technique improves awareness and helps to manage stress.

III. Integrating Somatic Practices into Daily Life:

1. Movement Breaks: Take brief movement breaks throughout the day. Stand upright, stretch, and move your body lightly. These pauses not only relieve physical strain but also improve cerebral clarity and attention.

2. Mindful Walking: Transform your everyday walks into mindfulness activities. Pay attention to each stride, the feel of your feet on the ground, and the rhythm of your breathing. This turns a normal task into a physical sensation.

3. *Evening Relaxation Routine*: Relax in the evening by following a somatic relaxation program. Calming exercises, progressive muscle relaxation, or a body scan meditation may help you release stress and prepare for a good night's sleep.

Breaking away from standard calorie formulae does not imply a rejection of scientific principles, but rather an acceptance of the limits of reductionist thinking in the context of holistic well-being. The somatic approach to weight control takes people on a deep journey—one that goes beyond numerical concerns and embraces the knowledge of the body-mind link. Individuals who prioritize mindful eating, stress management, and holistic well-being are on a long-term road that benefits both their bodies and brains.

Somatic practices evolve into partners on a lifetime journey of self-discovery, resilience, and empowered living, rather than just weight-management techniques. Individuals discover liberation in somatic weight control, which frees them from the confines of calorie monitoring and leads them into a more intuitive, balanced, and conscious living. It is a journey that goes beyond the numbers on a scale, enabling people to embrace the richness of the physical experience and create a harmonious connection with their bodies—one that endures and transcends diet culture's transient fads.

3.2 Adopting Holistic Health Practices to Maintain Well-Being

In the quest for well-being, a paradigm change is occurring that goes beyond the limiting limitations of traditional health paradigms. Holistic health techniques are becoming more popular as people seek overall well-being that includes physical, mental, emotional, and spiritual elements. This chapter delves into the fundamentals of holistic health, including how it promotes long-term well-being.

3.2.1 The Holistic Paradigm:

Holistic health differs from the reductionist approach, which divides the body into discrete components and focuses on symptoms rather than the underlying reasons for imbalance. At its foundation, holistic health recognizes the interdependence of many parts of a person's life, acknowledging that physical health, mental well-being, emotional balance, and spiritual satisfaction are all intertwined in a tapestry of completeness.

I. Principles of Holistic Health:

1. Interconnectedness: Holistic health holds that no component of a person acts alone. Physical health affects mental well-being, emotions influence the body, and spiritual satisfaction adds to total vitality.

Recognizing these interrelated processes is the cornerstone of holistic health.

2. *Individuality:* Holistic health recognizes the uniqueness of each individual. It considers a variety of elements, including heredity, lifestyle, environment, and personal experiences, recognizing that optimum well-being is a journey that is unique to each individual.

3. *Prevention and Balance*: Rather than concentrating exclusively on symptoms, holistic health emphasizes prevention and restoration of balance. This proactive approach tries to treat imbalances before they cause sickness and promotes the body's natural ability to repair itself.

4. *Mind-Body-Spirit Integration*: Holistic health emphasizes the interconnectedness of the mind, body, and spirit. It promotes activities that bring these aspects together, promoting a state of balance that goes beyond physical health to include mental clarity and spiritual harmony.

II. Holistic Health Approaches

1. Diet as Medicine: Holistic health emphasizes the importance of diet in total well-being. Rather than considering food just as fuel, holistic methods take into account the nourishing and healing effects of complete, nutrient-dense meals. Personalized nutrition strategies cater to individual requirements, promoting prolonged energy, immunological function, and bright health.

2. Mindfulness and Stress Reduction: Practices that promote awareness and decrease stress are essential for overall health. Mindfulness meditation, yoga, and other somatic methods include both the mind and the body, fostering relaxation, mental clarity, and emotional equilibrium. These activities promote overall well-being by addressing the linked effects of stress on physical, mental, and emotional health.

3. *Movement for Vitality:* Holistic health promotes regular physical activity that extends beyond the conventional definition of exercise. Tai chi, qigong, and somatic activities all improve physical fitness while also promoting energy flow, balance, and mental concentration. These exercises help to maintain well-being by boosting overall energy.

4. *Emotional Intelligence and Expression:* Holistic health emphasizes the importance of emotions in overall well-being. Journaling, expressive arts, and therapy are examples of practices that improve emotional intelligence. They help people negotiate and express their feelings. This emotional awareness helps to maintain mental and emotional equilibrium, which promotes long-term well-being.

5. *Integrative Medicine:* Holistic health promotes integrative techniques that mix traditional and alternative therapy. Integrative medicine focuses on the underlying causes of health problems, often combining standard medical procedures with techniques such as acupuncture, herbal medicine, and mind-body therapy. This holistic approach promotes long-term well-being by taking into account the full individual.

3.2.2 Holistic Health and Long-Term Well-being

I. Physical Well-being:

Holistic health methods focus on physical well-being by addressing the fundamentals of health, such as diet, exercise, and preventative treatment. Recognizing the body's innate capacity to heal and maintain balance allows people to embrace long-term behaviors that promote optimum physical health.

1. Nutrition for Longevity: Holistic health encourages a well-balanced, whole-foods-based diet that promotes both immediate and long-term health. Nutrient-dense meals provide vital vitamins, minerals, and antioxidants that promote cellular health, immunological function, and sustained energy.

2. Movement as a Lifelong Practice: Rather than perceiving exercise as a temporary fix, holistic health encourages people to see movement as a lifelong practice. Walking, yoga, and dancing are examples of delightful physical well-being activities.

3. Preventive Care and Holistic Check-Ins: Holistic health stresses frequent check-ins and preventive treatment to preserve physical health. Screenings, functional medicine exams, and holistic consultations are all examples of integrative health assessments that assist people uncover possible imbalances before they get unwell.

II. Mental Well-being:

Holistic health acknowledges the complex interaction between the mind and the body and understands that mental well-being is an essential component of long-term health. Individuals may nurture long-term mental health by including habits that promote mental clarity, emotional resilience, and psychological equilibrium.

1. Mindfulness Techniques for Mental Clarity: Holistic health advocates mindfulness techniques, such as meditation and focused breathing, to build mental clarity. These techniques provide people with strategies for managing stress, improving attention, and navigating the difficulties of contemporary life with resilience.

2. Emotional Resilience and Coping Strategies:
Holistic methods emphasize emotional intelligence
and resilience. Journaling and therapy treatments,
for example, help people build appropriate coping
mechanisms for life's obstacles, resulting in
long-term mental health.

3. Holistic Mental Health Support: Integrative
mental health treatments, such as psychotherapy,
counseling, and mind-body therapies, approach
mental health from a comprehensive standpoint.
These techniques promote long-term mental health
by taking into account the interconnections of
mental, emotional, and physical well-being.

III. Emotional Balance:

Emotional equilibrium, according to holistic health,
is a foundation of general well-being. Practices that
encourage self-awareness, emotional expression,
and good coping methods help to maintain
emotional balance.

1. *Expressive Arts and Creativity:* Holistic health acknowledges the therapeutic use of expressive arts in creating emotional equilibrium. Participating in creative activities such as painting, music, or dancing enables people to express and process their feelings, which promotes emotional well-being.

2. *Mind-Body Practices for Emotional Integration:* Holistic health incorporates mind-body practices, such as somatic exercises and body-centered treatments, to help in emotional integration. These techniques help people connect with and release emotions held in their bodies, resulting in a more balanced emotional state.

3. *Cultivating Healthy Relationships*: Fostering healthy relationships and social connections is part of a holistic approach to emotional health. Supportive connections provide emotional nutrition, foster a feeling of belonging, and are essential for maintaining emotional equilibrium.

IV. Spiritual Fulfillment:

Holistic health recognizes spiritual satisfaction as a component of complete well-being. While spirituality is a very individualized and unique component of human experience, activities that are consistent with individual beliefs and values help to maintain spiritual well-being.

1. Mindful Awareness and Presence: Holistic health promotes behaviors that foster mindfulness and presence. Mindfulness meditation, prayer, and contemplative activities help people connect with a deeper sense of purpose and spirituality.

2. Connection to Nature: Many holistic health systems highlight the healing relationship between people and nature. Spending time in nature, participating in outdoor activities, and admiring the beauty of the natural world all contribute to a feeling of spiritual contentment.

3. *Exploring Unique Beliefs*: Holistic health encourages people to discover and align with their unique beliefs. Individuals may cultivate a feeling of purpose and spiritual well-being by knowing what is meaningful in their lives.

3.2.3 Implementing Holistic Health Practices

This section offers practical advice for anyone wishing to adopt holistic health practices for long-term well-being.

1. *Personalized Well-Being Plan:* Create a customized well-being plan that includes holistic practices tailored to your specific requirements and interests. Consider things like diet, exercise, stress reduction, and emotional well-being.

2. *Holistic Health Assessments:* Check your whole health regularly, taking into account your physical, mental, emotional, and spiritual well-being. Holistic health exams may help you discover areas for improvement and promote long-term well-being.

3. *Integration of Holistic Practices:* Integrate holistic techniques into your everyday routine. This might include mindful eating, regular activity, moments of awareness throughout the day, and activities that are consistent with your spiritual beliefs. Consistent integration promotes overall well-being.

4. *Holistic Support Network:* Cultivate a support network that values holistic health ideas. Engage with others who have similar well-being objectives, get advice from integrative health specialists, and create a community to support your holistic path.

Embracing holistic health practices for long-term well-being is a never-ending quest. It is a continuing investigation of the linked elements of health—physical, mental, emotional, and spiritual. As people incorporate holistic practices into their lives, they begin on a journey that recognizes the wisdom of the body-mind-spirit connection.

Sustaining well-being via holistic health entails cultivating resilience, equilibrium, and a lasting feeling of energy. It is an invitation to live truthfully, by one's ideals, and create a healthy connection with oneself and the world. Individuals who embark on this holistic path not only improve their health, but also discover a deep feeling of purpose, pleasure, and satisfaction that will carry them through life's ups and downs.

CHAPTER 4: GENTLE MOVEMENTS, PROFOUND RESULTS

4.1 Gentle Exercises: Improving Posture, Flexibility, And Core Strength

Somatic exercise focuses on soft movements, providing a revolutionary approach to improving posture, flexibility, and core strength. This chapter digs into the importance of gentle exercises, examining how they contribute to general well-being and offering practical tips for implementing these motions into everyday routines.

4.1.1 The Essence of Gentle Exercise

Gentle exercises are the foundation of somatic practices, expressing a philosophy that values attentive movement above harsh effort. Unlike high-impact or hard workouts, gentle exercises emphasize fluidity, breath awareness, and muscular engagement. This technique not only provides physical advantages, but it also adheres to the principles of somatic exercise, improving the mind-body connection and total holistic health.

4.1.2 Understanding Posture, Flexibility, and Core Strength:

1. Posture: Posture is important for general health and well-being. Maintaining an appropriate spine and supporting structures reduces pressure on muscles and joints, improves breathing, and boosts mood and energy levels.

2. Flexibility: Flexibility is the ability of muscles and joints to move across their whole range of motion. Improved flexibility supports joint health, lowers the chance of injury, and increases general mobility. It is an essential part of effective mobility and somatic well-being.

3. Core Strength: The muscles in the belly, back, and pelvis provide a solid foundation for movement. Core strength improves balance, supports the spine, and is essential for many daily tasks, including sitting, standing, and walking.

4.1.3 The Benefits of Gentle Exercise

1. Mind-Body Connection: Gentle exercises are particularly effective in developing a strong mind-body connection. These exercises promote mindfulness by focusing on awareness of movement, breath, and sensations. This increased awareness not only improves the efficiency of the workouts but also extends to regular activities, encouraging mindful living.

2. Stress Reduction: The soft, rhythmic quality of these activities triggers a relaxation response in the neural system. Controlled breathing, mild stretching, and muscular relaxation may all help to reduce stress. This component is consistent with the wider somatic concept of treating the effects of stress on the body-mind link.

3. *Improved Posture:* Gentle activities naturally improve posture. By focusing on muscles that contribute to good alignment, these routines help people become more aware of their body's orientation. Muscle strengthening and lengthening occur gradually and contribute to long-term postural improvement.

4. *Enhanced Flexibility:* Gentle exercises are extremely beneficial in increasing flexibility. These workouts promote muscle lengthening and joint mobility by using slow, deliberate motions and stretches. This increased flexibility not only increases general mobility but also lowers the risk of injuries caused by stiffness and limited movement.

5. *Core Stability:* Many mild workouts are designed to improve core strength. These exercises activate the muscles that support the spine and pelvis, resulting in increased core stability. Core strength improves posture, serves as a basis for many physical activities, and protects against back problems.

4.1.4 Practical Ideas for Incorporating Gentle Exercises

I. Morning Mindful Movement Routine:

Objective: Start the day with easy movements to awaken the body and encourage a happy mood.

Routine:

- Start with deep, diaphragmatic breathing to calm the mind and oxygenate the body.
- To relieve stress, gently lengthen your neck by turning your head in each direction.

- Perform shoulder rolls, moving them forward and backward to relieve stiffness.
- Gradually advance to spine stretches, which include forward bends and twists.
- Use slow, controlled motions for the wrists and ankles to increase joint mobility.
- Finish with a few minutes of mindful standing while concentrating on grounding and centering.

II. Stress-Busting Breaks:

Objective: To fight the effects of stress, include short, stress-reducing workouts into your everyday routine.

Routine:

- For a few minutes, practice diaphragmatic breathing by inhaling deeply with your nose and gently expelling through your mouth.

- Incorporate sitting stretches that target areas of stress, such as the neck, shoulders, and lower back.

- Do mild sitting twists, To alleviate spinal tension.

- Take mindful walking breaks, paying attention to each step and cultivating a connection to the present moment.

III. Mindful Movement Throughout the Day:

Objective: Incorporate mindful movement into diverse tasks to encourage sustained involvement.

Integration:

- Incorporate seated stretches while working at a desk, focusing on neck, shoulders, and back.

- Use transitions between jobs to practice mild motions like wrist circles or ankle rolls.

- Practice mindful walking during breaks or on short outdoor walks, paying attention to each step.
- Incorporate standing stretches when waiting in line or taking brief breaks, emphasizing spine elongation.

IV. Evening Relaxation Routine:

Objective: End the day with easy movements to relieve stress and prepare the body for a good night's sleep.

Routine:

- Start with deep, soothing breathwork to communicate the body's transition to a relaxed state.
- Incorporate mild stretches throughout the body, concentrating on areas of stiffness or pain.

- Practice restorative yoga positions, holding them for a few minutes to promote relaxation.
- Finish with a body scan meditation, paying attention to each area of your body and releasing any leftover tension.

Incorporating mild exercises to enhance posture, flexibility, and core strength is more than just a physical regimen; it is a comprehensive approach to health. Individuals who practice mindful movement not only improve their physical fitness but also develop a stronger connection with their body. This chapter acts as a guide, encouraging people to investigate the transforming benefits of gentle exercises and incorporate them into their everyday lives to maintain somatic well-being.

In the ever-changing world of fitness and well-being, the paradigm of somatic movement modalities has gained popularity due to its holistic approach to improving physical and mental awareness. Among the many different somatic disciplines, three stand out for their distinct ideologies and transforming effects: Feldenkrais, BodyMind Centering, and Pilates. This chapter goes into the concepts and practices of each modality, providing a thorough examination of their contributions to somatic education and general well-being.

4.2.1 Feldenkrais Method:

I. Principles of the Feldenkrais Method:
Developed by Moshe Feldenkrais, the Feldenkrais Method is anchored on the idea that greater

awareness of movement patterns leads to better physical functioning and mental well-being. The technique has two main approaches: Awareness Through Movement (ATM) and Functional Integration.

1. *Awareness Through Movement (ATM):* This group-based technique combines verbal instructions and guided movements to encourage participants to experiment with different patterns while paying attention to feeling and awareness. The focus is on increasing self-awareness and improving movement quality rather than reaching particular goals.

2. *Functional Integration (FI):* In contrast, FI is a one-on-one session in which a practitioner guides an individual through tailored exercises using gentle touch and verbal prompts. The purpose is to address individual requirements and patterns, promoting better coordination and ease of movement.

II. Key Practices:

1. Mindful Exploration of Movement: Feldenkrais invites people to explore movement with a higher level of awareness. Slow, methodical sequences teach participants to recognize habitual patterns, uncover sources of stress, and explore new options for efficient and harmonious movement.

2. Variability and Adaptability: The technique promotes movement variability. Individuals may improve their adaptability and lower their risk of injury by experimenting with different motions and avoiding inflexible routines. This emphasis on unpredictability leads to greater flexibility and overall physical resilience.

3. Non-Judgmental Observation: Feldenkrais promotes nonjudgmental observation of one's movement. Participants are instructed to observe sensations, explore options without self-criticism, and progressively perfect their motions. This method encourages a positive and curious attitude toward one's body and skills.

4.2.2 BodyMind Centering:

I. Principles of BodyMind Centering:

Bonnie Bainbridge Cohen developed BodyMind Centering (BMC), which combines somatic psychology, developmental movement patterns, and embodied anatomy. The modality uses experiential movement and hands-on approaches to investigate the link between the body, mind, and consciousness.

1. Embodied Anatomy: BMC emphasizes embodied anatomy, which involves experiencing and comprehending anatomy via movement and direct sensory experience. This technique enables people to investigate the functioning and interactions of many bodily systems in a holistic and embodied manner.

2. *Developmental Movement Patterns:* BMC takes influence from developing movement patterns seen in early human development. Participants participate in movements that correspond to developmental stages, developing a strong connection with underlying patterns that form both physical and psychological aspects of being.

3. *Bodily System Integration:* This modality investigates the interconnection of bodily systems while also understanding the impact of emotions, thoughts, and experiences on physical functioning. Individuals get a comprehensive awareness of the dynamic interaction between many parts of the body and mind via guided experiences.

II. Key Practices:

1. Experiential Anatomy Classes: At BMC, participants typically participate in guided movement explorations to get a better knowledge of anatomical structures and functions. This hands-on method increases body awareness and fosters a tactile knowledge of anatomy.

2. Developmental Movement Exploration: Participants take part in movement sequences inspired by developmental patterns, engaging with the underlying knowledge embedded in their bodies' developmental history. This investigation attempts to raise awareness of fundamental motions that underpin more sophisticated actions.

3. Hands-On Bodywork: In BMC, hands-on bodywork is used to assist people in discovering their movement patterns. Touch and verbal cues are used by practitioners to help people feel more embodied, release tension, and move more seamlessly and efficiently.

4.2.3 Pilates:

I. Principles of Pilates:

Joseph Pilates developed Pilates, a mind-body training regimen that improves strength, flexibility, and general physical health. Pilates revolves around the idea of a strong core, often known as the "powerhouse," which encompasses the muscles of the belly, lower back, hips, and buttocks.

1. Core Engagement: Pilates focuses on activating and developing the core muscles. Movements start from the core, fostering stability, balance, and general postural alignment. This emphasis on core activation leads to increased bodily awareness and control.

2. Precision and Control: Pilates stresses accuracy in movement execution and control throughout each exercise. Practitioners are advised to focus on alignment, breathing, and movement quality, which promotes a conscious and purposeful approach to exercise.

3. Breath Integration: Breathing is an essential part of Pilates workouts. Coordinating breath and movement improves oxygenation, core engagement, and general relaxation and attention. The integration of breath promotes a comprehensive experience that links the mind and body.

II. Key Practices:

1. Mat-Based and Equipment-Based Exercises: Pilates provides several exercises that may be done on a mat or with specialist equipment such as the Reformer, Cadillac, and Wunda Chair. Mat-based workouts utilize your body weight as resistance, while equipment-based exercises employ spring resistance to challenge and support the body.

2. Progressive Sequences: Pilates movements are often designed in progressive sequences that steadily increase in intensity and complexity. This strategy helps people to gradually increase their strength, endurance, and flexibility, making it suitable for practitioners of all fitness levels.

3. Mindful Movement Flow: Pilates promotes a fluid and continuous movement flow between exercises. This emphasis on fluidity aids with coordination, balance, and heightened body awareness during transitions between moves.

4.2.4 Integrating Somatic Modalities for Holistic Well-Being

I. Complementary Aspects of Feldenkrais, BodyMind Centering, and Pilates

While Feldenkrais, BodyMind Centering, and Pilates all have their own set of concepts and practices, certain overlaps lead to a more holistic approach to wellness.

1. Mind-Body Connection: All three techniques stress the significance of the mind-body link. Whether via mindful movement explorations (Feldenkrais), experiential anatomy (BodyMind Centering), or precise control (Pilates), practitioners are encouraged to create awareness and presence in their movements.

2. Individualized Discovery: Each modality promotes individual discovery and adaptation. Individuals may adjust practices to their requirements, whether they are investigating variations in movement patterns (Feldenkrais), embracing developmental sequences (BodyMind Centering), or developing via tailored workouts (Pilates).

3. *Breath Awareness:* Each of the three methods focuses on breath. Whether via conscious breathing during movement (Feldenkrais), examining breath as an intrinsic aspect of movement (BodyMind Centering), or precisely controlling breath (Pilates), breath integration improves the whole somatic experience.

Exploring somatic movement modalities (Feldenkrais, BodyMind Centering, and Pilates) uncovers a tapestry of somatic knowledge that addresses the complexities of human experience. Each method promotes holistic well-being by encouraging people to interact with their bodies, increase awareness, and recognize the interdependence of physical and mental health.

By adopting these somatic activities into their everyday lives, people may improve their movement quality, encourage self-discovery, and get a better knowledge of their embodied existence. Individuals may weave various somatic modalities into a rich and transforming path toward holistic well-being, whether they want to explore movement gently, get embodied knowledge from developmental patterns, or improve their accuracy and strength with core-focused exercises.

CHAPTER 5: BREATHWORK FOR WEIGHT HARMONY

5.1 Understanding the Interconnectedness of Breathing, Metabolism, and Emotional Regulation

In the complicated dance of human physiology, the interconnectivity of breath, metabolism, and emotional regulation has a significant impact on our general well-being. This chapter delves into the complex links between these three essential characteristics of human functioning, offering light on how their harmony affects not only our physical health but also our emotional moods and mental balance.

5.1.1 The Breath:

I. Physiology of Breathing:

Breathing is a key physiological mechanism that goes beyond only oxygen exchange. The respiratory system is essential for maintaining the body's acid-base balance and managing carbon dioxide levels, which influence blood pH. The diaphragm, a main muscle involved in breathing, not only allows for air intake but also communicates with the neurological system, regulating our stress response.

II. Breath and Nervous System:

The breath bridges the gap between the neurological system's voluntary and involuntary functions. Conscious control over breathing, as shown in activities such as deep diaphragmatic breathing or pranayama, may activate the parasympathetic nerve system, facilitating relaxation and mitigating the stress response. Conversely, shallow or quick breathing may activate the sympathetic nervous system, resulting in increased arousal and tension.

5.1.2 Metabolism:

I. Metabolic processes:

Metabolism refers to the complicated metabolic processes that convert food into energy, which supports a variety of physiological tasks. The basal metabolic rate (BMR) is the amount of energy used during rest to sustain fundamental body activities. Metabolism is regulated by genetics, body composition, and physical activity, demonstrating the dynamic nature of energy balance in the organism.

II. Hormone Regulation and Metabolism:

Hormones have an important function in metabolic control. The pancreas produces insulin, which stimulates glucose absorption by cells for energy generation. Cortisol, which is often linked with stress, may affect metabolism by mobilizing energy reserves during fight-or-flight reactions. Thyroid hormones control the metabolic rate, which influences energy consumption and heat generation.

5.1.3 Emotional Regulation:

I. Emotional Responses and Autonomic Nervous System:

Emotions are complex reactions that include physiological, psychological, and behavioral components. The autonomic nervous system, which includes sympathetic and parasympathetic branches, is responsible for coordinating emotional reactions. Stressful stimuli stimulate the sympathetic response, preparing the body for action, while relaxing activities activate the parasympathetic response, which promotes relaxation.

II. The Role of Neurotransmitters:

Neurotransmitters, or chemical messengers in the brain, help regulate emotions. Diet and sunshine exposure both affect serotonin, which is connected with mood stability. Dopamine, which is connected to pleasure and reward, may influence motivation and emotional well-being. Imbalances in neurotransmitter levels are linked to mood disorders such as sadness and anxiety.

5.1.4 Interplay:

I. Breath and Emotional Regulation:

The breath is a strong modulator of emotional moods. Mindful breathing practices, such as deep diaphragmatic breathing or coherent breathing, stimulate the parasympathetic nervous system, promoting relaxation and emotional equilibrium. Conscious control of the breath gives a practical tool for navigating and managing emotional reactions.

II. Breath and Metabolism:

The breath is inextricably related to metabolism via the gas exchange involved in cellular respiration. Efficient oxygen supply to cells promotes metabolic processes and influences energy generation. Optimizing breathing patterns improves metabolic efficiency, which may influence weight control and overall energy balance.

III. Metabolism and Emotional Regulation:

Metabolic processes help to regulate emotions by producing neurotransmitters and ensuring the availability of energy substrates. Blood glucose levels must remain stable to maintain mood stability since variations might influence emotional well-being. Physical exercise, a component of metabolism, is linked to the production of endorphins, which promote happy moods.

5.1.5 Practices for Harmony:

I. Mindful Breathing Exercises:

1. Diaphragmatic Breathing: Inhale deeply through the nose, allowing the diaphragm to expand before gently expelling through the mouth. This technique triggers the relaxation response and promotes emotional equilibrium.

2. Coherent Breathing: Inhale and exhale with equal durations, such as a count of four. This rhythmic breathing style increases heart rate variability while increasing emotional resilience and equilibrium.

II. Metabolism-Friendly Lifestyle Options:

1. Balanced Nutrition: Eat a healthy diet that promotes stable blood glucose levels. Use a balance of complex carbs, lean proteins, and healthy fats to give long-lasting energy and support metabolic functions.

2. *Physical Exercise:* Regular physical exercise promotes metabolic efficiency and mental well-being. Activities like walking, running, and yoga help to release endorphins, which promote a pleasant mood.

III. Integrative Practices:

1. *Breath-Centered Meditation:* Use breath-centered meditation techniques to improve awareness and emotional control. Focus on the breath as an anchor for awareness, allowing emotions to emerge and pass without judgment.

2. *Mindful Eating:* Enjoy each mouthful, pay attention to hunger and fullness signs, and cultivate a healthy connection with food. This strategy promotes mental health and metabolic balance.

The symphony of breath, metabolism, and emotional control creates a tapestry of well-being that transcends the boundaries of particular body systems. Understanding their interdependence encourages us to investigate holistic techniques that balance these aspects, promoting a state of harmony in which physical vitality, emotional resilience, and mental clarity coexist.

Individuals may achieve a holistic approach to well-being by practicing mindful breathing, supporting metabolic health via lifestyle choices, and establishing emotional regulation techniques. This journey is not a goal, but rather a continuous inquiry in which each breath, metabolic function, and emotional reaction adds to the symphony of a healthy and vibrant existence.

5.2 Practical Breathwork Techniques for Daily Integration and Weight Balance

In the search for holistic well-being, using practical breathwork methods has considerable promise for promoting emotional balance and weight control. This chapter looks at a variety of accessible and effective breathwork routines that may be easily incorporated into everyday living. Individuals may start on a path of self-discovery and increased vitality by combining breath's transforming potential with careful attention to weight balance.

5.2.1 Breath Awareness:

I. Mindful Breathing Observation:

Begin your path to practical breathwork by being aware of your normal breathing rhythm. Spend a few minutes observing the rise and fall of your breath. Consider the feeling of the breath as it enters and exits your body. This basic act of careful observation creates the groundwork for forming a conscious connection with your breath.

II. Diaphragmatic Breathing:

Diaphragmatic breathing, also known as abdominal or deep breathing, is a basic breathwork method that helps you relax and stimulates your parasympathetic nervous system. Take these steps:

1. Find a comfortable sitting or laying posture.
2. Put one hand on your chest, and the other on your belly.
3. Take deep breaths through your nose, allowing your abdomen to expand.
4. Slowly exhale through your lips while feeling your abdomen constrict.
5. Maintain this regular breathing while concentrating on the gradual rise and fall of your abdomen.

III. Coherent Breathing for Stress Relief:

Coherent breathing is a rhythmic breathing method that increases heart rate variability, promotes emotional resilience, and reduces stress. Perform the following cohesive breathing exercise:

1. Inhale for four counts.
2. Exhale to a count of four.
3. Continue this regular breathing pattern for a few minutes, ensuring a smooth and continuous flow.

IV. Box Breathing for Focus and Balance:

Box breathing, also known as square breathing, is a systematic breathwork method that helps with attention and balance. Follow this easy box-breathing sequence:

1. Inhale for four counts.
2. Hold your breath for four counts.
3. Exhale to a count of four.

4. Hold your breath for four counts.

5. Repeat this cycle numerous times, allowing each phase to flow smoothly into the next.

5.2.2 Breathing Exercises for Emotional Balance and Weight Management:

I. Breath of Fire for Energy Activation:

Breath of Fire is a dynamic and stimulating breathwork method that originated in Kundalini Yoga. It is characterized by rhythmic, fast breathing via the nose, with an emphasis on the exhale. This method stimulates the solar plexus, enhancing energy flow and producing a sensation of vigor.

1. Sit comfortably with an erect spine.

2. Inhale deeply through your nose.

3. Exhalation firmly and quickly through your nostrils, concentrating on the exhalation.

4. Allow the inhalation to come naturally while keeping your concentration on the strong exhale.

5. Repeat for 1-3 minutes, progressively increasing the length over time.

II. Nadi Shodhana for Balance:

Nadi Shodhana, or alternate nostril breathing, is a breathwork practice that balances the left and right hemispheres of the brain. This technique promotes tranquility and mental stability while improving general well-being.

1. Sit comfortably with an erect spine.

2. Close your right nostril with your thumb and take a deep breath in through your left.

3. Close your left nostril with your right ring finger, then exhale.

4. Inhale deeply via your right nostril.

5. Close the right nostril, open the left, and exhale.

6. Continue this alternate cycle for many minutes while keeping a steady and balanced breath.

5.2.3 Integrating Breathwork into Everyday Life:

I. Mindful Breathing Breaks:

Incorporate mindful breathing pauses into your everyday routine to increase your feeling of calm and presence. Set out a few minutes each day for deliberate breathwork, such as a round of coherent breathing, diaphragmatic breathing, or a short period of breath observation.

II. Breathing Awareness during Physical Activity:

Incorporate breath awareness into your physical activities like walking, running, and yoga. Coordinate your breath with your actions, allowing your breath's rhythm to lead and support you. This integration improves attention and fosters a comprehensive connection between the breath and the body.

III. Breath-Centered Meditation for Daily Reflections:

Practice breath-centered meditation as a method of daily introspection. Find a quiet area, sit comfortably, and concentrate on your breathing. Allow your breath to lead you into a state of inner calm, creating room for self-awareness, clarity, and focused reflection.

5.2.4 Weight Balance and Breathing:

I. Mindful Eating Practices:

Integrate breathwork into your mealtime routine. Before meals, spend a few seconds to focus yourself with diaphragmatic breathing. During meals, practice mindful breathing in between bites to increase awareness of hunger and fullness signals.

This method encourages a deliberate and balanced relationship with eating.

II. Breath as an Anchor for Emotional Resilience:
During emotional times, use your breath to anchor yourself. When stressed, anxious, or experiencing emotional swings, use coherent or diaphragmatic breathing. The purposeful concentration on your breath serves as a grounding factor, promoting emotional control and resilience.

The use of practical breathwork practices in everyday life provides a pathway to overall well-being, including emotional balance and weight control. By incorporating breath awareness into our daily lives, we get access to a reservoir of inner resilience and mindfulness.

Accept the simplicity and accessibility of breathwork and make it a daily companion on your road to balance. Whether it's the rhythmic coherence of your breath during a difficult situation or the deliberate diaphragmatic breath before a meal, the breath serves as a trustworthy anchor, creating a harmonious connection between mind, body, and emotions. As you begin this breath-centered inquiry, may each inhale and exhalation leads you to a more lively and balanced way of life.

CHAPTER 6: DEVELOPING MINDFUL EATING HABITS

6.1 Developing Habits for Conscious Food Choices and Portion Control

The decisions we make about food and the quantities we eat are critical components of our overall well-being. Cultivating habits that encourage mindful eating and portion management is essential not just for maintaining a healthy weight, but also for feeding our bodies and developing a pleasant connection with food. This chapter delves into successful tactics and practical ideas for developing habits that enable people to make thoughtful decisions and accept moderation in their eating patterns.

6.1.1 Conscious Food Choices:

I. Mindful Eating Philosophy:

At the heart of conscious food choices is the notion of mindful eating. This method encourages people to pay full attention and awareness to the present moment, enabling them to enjoy the sensory experience of eating, notice hunger and fullness signals, and make choices aligned with their overall well-being.

II. Breaking Free from Emotional Eating:

Emotional eating is a prevalent challenge often linked to stress, boredom, or other emotions. Recognizing and treating emotional triggers is an important part of developing habits for mindful eating. Practices such as journaling, deep breathing, and engaging in alternative activities can effectively disrupt the cycle of emotional eating.

6.1.2 Practical Strategies for Making Conscious Food Choices:

I. Menu Planning and Preparation:

1. Weekly Meal Planning: Set aside time each week to plan your meals. This technique not only promotes a well-balanced diet but also reduces impulsive eating selections.

2. Nutrient-Rich Ingredients: When planning your meals, prioritize nutrient-dense foods. To make balanced and fulfilling meals, include a mix of fruits, vegetables, whole grains, lean meats, and healthy fats.

II. Mindful Grocery Shopping:

1. Make a List: Before going to the grocery store, make a list based on your meal plans. Stick to the list to prevent making unplanned and perhaps unhealthy purchases.

2. Shop the Perimeter: The perimeter of the grocery store usually has fresh fruit, lean proteins, and dairy. Focus on these areas to promote full, unprocessed meals.

III. Portion Awareness:

1. Use Smaller Plates: Choose smaller plates to give the appearance of greater meals. This visual method might help you regulate portion sizes and avoid overeating.

2. Practice Portion Control: Be careful of serving sizes and resist the desire to go for seconds right away. Allow some time before determining whether you need extra food.

6.1.3 The Role of the Environment in Conscious Eating:

I. Create a Supportive Eating Environment:

1. Minimize Distractions: Create a relaxing and distraction-free dining atmosphere. Turn off your devices, sit at a table, and enjoy the sensory experience of dining.

2. Mindful Eating Rituals: Create mindful eating rituals, such as expressing thanks before meals or pausing to enjoy the colors and sensations of your food.

6.1.4 Building a Positive Relationship with Food:

I. Intuitive Eating Practices:

1. Listen to Hunger Cues: Pay attention to your body's hunger signals. Eat when you are hungry, and quit when you are full. This practice cultivates a more intuitive and sensitive attitude to eating.

2. Enjoy Treats Mindfully: Give yourself occasional treats without guilt. When indulging, appreciate each meal carefully, concentrating on the enjoyment of the experience.

6.1.5 Establishing Sustainable Habits:

I. Gradual Changes for Long-term Success:

1. Start Small: To prevent overwhelming oneself, implement adjustments gradually. Concentrate on one or two behaviors at a time until they become automatic components of your routine.

2. Consistency is Key: Consistency is critical in habit building. Aim for consistency in your mindful eating activities to reinforce beneficial behaviors over time.

II. Reflect and Adjust:

1. Reflection: Review your eating patterns regularly. Determine what works well and what may need improvement. Be willing to adjust your strategy in response to changing circumstances.

2. Seek Support: Share your experience with friends, family, or a support group. A supportive community may provide encouragement and accountability.

Developing habits for Conscious food choices and portion management is a step toward adopting a mindful nutrition lifestyle. Individuals who incorporate these tactics into their every day lives may establish a healthy connection with food, improve their general health, and achieve long-term weight control.

As you begin on this journey, keep in mind that each decision adds to the bigger picture of your well-being. Whether it's the deliberate choice of nutrient-dense meals, the practice of portion awareness, or the establishment of a supportive eating environment, these habits weave together to produce a tapestry of mindful living—one in which nutrition, satisfaction, and balance live together.

May your path be led by the wisdom of deliberate decisions and the transformational power of mindful eating.

6.2 Liberating Yourself from Emotional Eating Cycles

Because of the complex interaction between emotions and eating, many people get trapped in a cycle of emotional eating—a habit in which food acts as a coping technique for stress, melancholy, boredom, or other emotional states. To break free from this pattern, you must first raise your awareness, address any underlying emotional triggers, and develop healthy coping methods. This chapter delves into the complexity of emotional eating, providing insights and practical solutions for breaking free from its grasp and promoting a more balanced and thoughtful attitude to food.

6.2.1 Understanding Emotional Eating:

I. Emotional Eating Connection:

Emotional eating is when people use food to calm, console, or repress their emotions. It typically goes beyond bodily hunger, fueled by a need for emotional comfort or diversion. Stress, worry, depression, loneliness, and even celebrations are common causes.

II. The Cycle of Emotional Eating:

1. Emotional Trigger: An emotional event or stressor causes an intense emotional reaction.

2. Food as Comfort: To deal with their emotions, people resort to food for comfort and diversion.

3. Temporary Relief: Eating offers a brief feeling of comfort or pleasure, but it does not treat the underlying emotional problem.

4. Guilt and Regret: Following consumption, emotions of guilt and regret may emerge, resulting in a downward emotional cycle.

5. *Repetition:* The cycle repeats, cementing the link between emotion and eating.

6.2.2 Developing Awareness:

I. Mindful Observation of Triggers:

Developing awareness is the first step toward freedom from emotional eating. Pay attention to the circumstances, feelings, or events that cause you to eat emotionally. Keep a notebook to document these incidents, noting the emotions involved and the foods selected.

II. Distinguishing Physical from Emotional Hunger:

Learn the difference between physical and emotional hunger. Physical hunger usually develops gradually and is satiated with a range of meals. Emotional hunger, on the other hand, is characterized by sudden, particular cravings for comfort foods. Before grabbing for food, think about how hungry you are.

6.2.3 Strategies for Breaking the Cycle:

I. Developing Healthy Coping Mechanisms:

1. Emotional Awareness Practices: Try mindfulness meditation, deep breathing exercises, or journaling. These strategies provide a place for understanding and processing emotions without relying on food.

2. Physical Exercise: Include regular physical exercise in your daily routine. Exercise not only increases endorphins, which improve mood, but it also gives an outlet for stress and emotions.

II. Building a Support System:

1. Share Your Journey: Talk to friends, relatives, or a support group about your emotional eating issues. Sharing your story builds a supportive network and alleviates feelings of loneliness.

2. *Seek Professional Guidance:* Consider seeing a therapist or counselor. Professional treatment may help you resolve deeper emotional problems and develop coping methods that are suited to your specific requirements.

6.2.4 Mindful Eating Practices:

I. Conscious Food Choices:

1. *Take a Moment Before Eating*: Prior to grabbing a meal, pause to assess your emotional state. Consider if you're eating out of actual hunger or in reaction to emotions.

2. *Choose Nutrient-Dense meals*: When emotional hunger strikes, go for nutrient-dense meals that will replenish your body. Add colorful fruits and vegetables, lean meats, and healthy grains to your meals.

II. Mindful-Eating Techniques:

1. Savor Each Meal: Slow down your eating rate and enjoy each meal. Concentrate on the tastes, textures, and feelings of the meal. This practice improves the awareness of eating.

2. Eat Without Distractions: Remove all distractions to create a concentrated dining atmosphere. Turn off your devices, sit down at a table, and engage in the process of dining.

6.2.5 Rewriting the Narrative:

I. Shifting Perceptions about Food:

1. Let Go of Food Guilt: Release any guilt linked to emotional eating. Recognize that food is a source of sustenance and that occasional indulgences are an acceptable element of a healthy eating regimen.

2. Reframe Emotional Responses: Consider other methods to deal with emotions. Instead of resorting to food for consolation, try doing something that makes you happy, relaxed, or fulfilled.

II. Self-Compassion Practices:

1. Practice Self-Compassion: Take a sympathetic attitude towards oneself. Recognize that everyone encounters obstacles, and self-compassion is vital for breaking away from the pattern of emotional eating.

2. Appause Progress: Recognize and applaud tiny accomplishments along the road. Celebrating achievement encourages a good attitude and supports attempts to address emotional eating tendencies.

Liberating oneself from emotional eating cycles is a transforming path that begins with self-awareness, conscious choices, and compassionate self-care. Individuals may interrupt the pattern of emotional eating by identifying their triggers, establishing healthy coping methods, and cultivating a good connection with food. Remember that emancipation is about progress, not perfection. Each step toward mindful eating and emotional awareness brings you closer to a better, more balanced relationship with food. May your journey be marked by self-compassion, resilience, and the powerful awareness that you can break free from emotional eating and embrace a more rewarding and healthy way of life.

CHAPTER 7: CREATING A PERSONALIZED SOMATIC ROUTINE

7.1 Developing a Sustainable Somatic Exercise Practice for Your Lifestyle

In the world of wellness, somatic exercise develops as a comprehensive strategy that goes beyond standard fitness regimens. Somatic exercises aim to engage the mind-body connection, increase awareness, and promote fluid movement patterns. Designing a sustainable somatic exercise practice that is adapted to your lifestyle entails a careful integration of these concepts, ensuring that the benefits of this attentive approach flow easily into your everyday life.

7.1.1 Understanding Somatic Exercise:

I. Embracing Mindful Movement:

Somatic exercise is based on the notion of conscious movement, which emphasizes the relationship between body and mind. Unlike traditional workouts, which typically emphasize exterior outcomes, somatic exercises focus on the interior experience of movement, urging people to be present and sensitive to the feelings in their bodies.

II. Principles of Somatic Exercise:

1. Body Awareness: Somatic exercises emphasize increased awareness of physical sensations, movements, and postures. This self-awareness lays the groundwork for developing a stronger relationship with your body.

2. Gentle Exploration: Somatic movement is defined by gentle, inquisitive gestures. Somatic exercises promote a gentler and more adaptive approach to movement, rather than forcing the body to do rigid or aggressive activities.

3. *Tension Release:* One of the most important aspects of somatic exercise is releasing excess tension from the muscles. Individuals may enhance their flexibility and lessen their pain by focusing on tight regions and allowing them to relax.

7.1.2   Tailoring Somatic Exercise for Your Lifestyle:

I. Assessing Your Schedule and Preferences:

1. *Time Commitment:* Consider your daily routine and how much time you can reasonably devote to somatic exercise. Whether it's brief sessions throughout the day or lengthier practices a few times a week, finding a balance that fits your schedule is critical.

2. Preferred Modalities: Experiment with somatic exercise modalities including Feldenkrais, BodyMind Centering, and Pilates. Each modality provides a distinct approach to movement and body awareness. Choose the one that most closely matches your tastes and aims.

II. Integrating Somatic Exercises into Everyday Activities:

1. Micro-Movements: Add micro-movements to your routine. These modest, purposeful motions may be smoothly incorporated into activities such as standing, walking, and sitting. They gradually increase body awareness and minimize muscle stress.

2. Mindful Transitions: Pay attention to the transitions between tasks. Use these opportunities to do short somatic exercises, enabling your body to reset and release any collected tension before on to the next job.

7.1.3 Designing Your Personalized Somatic Exercise Routine:

I. Warm-Up and Centering:

1. Body Scan: Start with a body scan to identify any points of tension or pain. This helps provide the groundwork for focused and mindful movement.

2. Breath Awareness: Focus on your breathing. Before beginning somatic activities, diaphragmatic breathing may help you center yourself and develop a feeling of presence.

II. Gentle Movements to Improve Posture and Flexibility:

1. Joint Articulation: Use mild joint articulation exercises to lubricate and mobilize your joints. This might involve motions for the neck, shoulders, spine, hips, and ankles, which improve general flexibility.

2. *Cat-Cow Stretch:* Move between arched and rounded postures to increase spinal flexibility and relieve back stress.

III. Mindful Exploration of Movement Modalities:

1. *Feldenkrais Explorations:* Incorporate Feldenkrais concepts by doing exploratory movements. Concentrate on small differences and observe how your body reacts to various motion patterns.

2. *BodyMind Centering Practices:* Use BodyMind Centering techniques that stress the relationship between bodily systems and sensations. This might include mild motions that correspond to the breath and enhance general well-being.

IV. Breath-Centered Integration:

1. *Coordinated Breath and Movement:* Make sure your breath and movement match. Synchronize inhales with expanding motions, and exhales with contracting ones. This conscious integration improves the mind-body link.

2. Breath Expansion Activities: Perform breath expansion activities to encourage deep diaphragmatic breathing. This might include completely breathing and stretching your ribcage, which allows for better oxygenation and relaxation.

IV. Closing and Integration:

1. Body Scan Revisited: Finish your somatic workout regimen with a body scan to target areas of stress. Make a note of any changes in feeling or locations where you feel more open and relaxed.

2. Gratitude and Reflection: Express thanks for the time you've spent on your somatic practice. Reflect on the feelings and insights you got throughout the session, keeping a good attitude.

7.1.4 Overcoming Challenges and Maintaining Motivation:

I. Common Challenges of Somatic Exercise:

1. Patience and Persistence: Somatic exercises often need patience and perseverance. Results may not be immediately visible, therefore it is critical to approach the practice with a long-term mindset.

2. Adapting to Changes: As your body changes, so should your somatic exercise regimen. Be willing to adjust and change movements depending on your changing requirements and experiences.

II. Motivational Strategies:

1. Set Realistic Goals: Create attainable objectives that are consistent with your overall well-being. Setting realistic expectations promotes motivation, whether it is for more flexibility, less muscle tension, or increased body awareness.

2. Connect with a Community: Participating in a somatic exercise community or taking a somatic movement class gives a feeling of belonging and support. Sharing your experiences and views with others helps boost motivation and accountability.

Designing a sustained somatic exercise practice that fits your lifestyle is an opportunity to embrace the flexibility of conscious movement. Somatic exercises become a way of life when they are consciously integrated into everyday activities, tailored routines, and a dedication to overcoming problems. Keep in mind that somatic exercise is a constantly developing discipline. Your body's requirements, preferences, and reactions will direct your journey. May the gentle study of somatic movement bring you pleasure, vigor, and overall well-being—a transforming journey that is easily integrated into your everyday life.

Finding time for dedicated workouts might be difficult in today's fast-paced lifestyle. However, the concept of fitness goes beyond a gym or an organized workout regimen. Individuals may develop persistent involvement with physical activity by smoothly incorporating exercises into their everyday lives, improving overall well-being, and removing the hurdles associated with conventional workouts.

7.2.1 Recognize the Need for Consistent Engagement:

I. Impact of Daily Movement:
Consistent physical exercise has significant consequences for general health. Regular exercise has several advantages, including improved cardiovascular fitness, increased physical strength,

136

and mental well-being. The idea is to reframe exercise as an integrated and continuous element of everyday life rather than a discrete, time-bound activity.

II. Breaking Down Barriers:

Traditional impediments to exercise, such as a lack of time, desire, or access to a gym, might prevent frequent participation. Integrating workouts into everyday living eliminates these obstacles, making physical activity more accessible and realistic for people with a variety of lives and responsibilities.

7.2.2 Unveiling Opportunities for Integration:

I. Embracing Everyday Movements:

1. Active Commuting: Use active forms of transportation, such as walking or cycling, wherever practical. If your employment is reasonably close, try combining these things into your regular commute.

2. *Stair Utilization:* Use Stairs Instead of Elevators or Escalators. Climbing stairs is an excellent aerobic exercise that involves a variety of muscle groups, leading to increased fitness.

II. Microbreak Movements:

1. *Desk workouts:* Incorporate easy workouts into your workday routine. During brief intervals, do seated leg lifts, chair squats, or desk push-ups to energize your body and counteract the effects of extended sitting.

2. *Stretching Breaks:* Schedule stretching breaks throughout the day. Simple stretches may help relieve muscular tension, increase flexibility, and promote a more energetic and focused mentality.

III. Household Fitness Integration:

1. *Active Cleaning:* Turn domestic duties into exercise opportunities. Engage your core while cleaning, lunges while folding clothes, or squats while picking up objects off the floor.

2. Dance Breaks: Transform dull circumstances into dance breaks. Moving to music adds a joyful aspect to everyday duties, whether you're cooking, cleaning dishes, or waiting for the kettle to boil. It also provides cardiovascular advantages.

IV. Mindful Movement Practices:

1. Mindful Walking: Incorporate mindful walking into your everyday routines. Concentrate on the sensations of each step while keeping proper posture and using your muscles. This simple activity raises awareness and encourages a more thoughtful attitude to movement.

2. Breathwork Integration: Incorporate breathwork into regular activities. Practice diaphragmatic breathing when sitting in traffic, waiting in line, or under stress. This purposeful integration promotes relaxation and general well-being.

7.2.3 Designing Your Integrated Exercise Routine:

I. Personalized Planning:

1. Identify Time Pockets: Examine your daily calendar to locate time slots that lend themselves to physical exercise. This might include morning routines, lunch breaks, and nighttime rituals.

2. Set Realistic Goals: Set attainable fitness objectives that are compatible with your lifestyle. Setting realistic goals, whether it's a certain amount of steps per day or combining brief bursts of movement, improves long-term adherence.

II. Integrating Movement Modalities:

1. Diverse Workouts: Use a range of workouts to avoid boredom and adapt to diverse interests. For a more comprehensive approach, include aerobic activities, weight training, flexibility exercises, and balancing drills into your daily regimen.

2. *Somatic Practices*: Include somatic activities in your everyday routine. Practice mindful movement with a focus on body awareness, gentle exploration, and tension release. Somatic exercises integrate easily into everyday activities, promoting a healthy connection between mind and body.

III. Accountability and Tracking:

1. *Activities Tracking:* Use fitness trackers or apps to track your daily activities. Tracking allows you to see your progress, recognize your accomplishments, and keep on track with your fitness objectives.

2. *Accountability Partners:* Enlist a friend or family member as an exercise partner. Shared commitment and encouragement boost motivation, increasing the likelihood that both persons will maintain a regular level of physical exercise.

7.2.4 Overcoming Challenges and Maintaining Motivation:

I. Addressing Common Obstacles:

1. Time Management: Treat physical exercise as a vital element of your daily routine. Schedule exercise breaks just like any other appointment to build a feeling of commitment.

2. Adaptability: Include flexibility in your workout program. Life's unpredictability may necessitate changes, and being adaptive guarantees that you can easily incorporate physical exercise into shifting situations.

II. Motivational Strategies:

1. Celebrate Small Wins: Recognize and applaud modest victories in your fitness regimen.

Recognizing achievement, whether it's finishing a set of exercises or regularly hitting your daily step target, encourages a good attitude.

2. Incorporate Enjoyable Activities: Participate in activities that you like. Whether it's dancing, gardening, or playing sports, including delightful motions boosts motivation and turns exercise into a pleasurable experience.

Integrating workouts effortlessly into everyday life goes beyond the traditional limitations of fitness, resulting in a lifestyle in which movement is inherent to daily activities. Individuals may incorporate frequent physical exercise into their lives by identifying opportunities, tailoring routines, and overcoming obstacles. May this approach inspire you to adopt a lifestyle in which activity is not a chore but a vital and satisfying part of every day, leading to a healthier, more vibrant life.

CHAPTER 8: INTEGRATING SOMATICS AND NUTRITION

8.1 Synergies of Somatics and Nutrition for Holistic Weight Management

In the goal of comprehensive weight control, the junction of somatics and nutrition provides a potent synergy that goes beyond traditional methods. Somatics, with its emphasis on the mind-body connection and conscious movement, complements nutritional concepts to provide a complete framework for anyone seeking long-term and overall well-being. This chapter investigates the dynamic relationship between somatics and nutrition, emphasizing how integrating these two pillars might lead to a more balanced and transformational path toward holistic weight control.

8.1.1 Understanding the Foundation:

I. Somatics:

Somatics refers to a variety of disciplines that emphasize the connection of the mind and body. Somatics allows people to discover and comprehend their bodies' unique language via gentle movements, breathwork, and increased body awareness. This technique goes beyond typical fitness, stressing the value of developing a mindful and intuitive connection with one's physical body.

II. Nutrition:

Nutrition, on the other hand, offers the necessary building blocks for the body's proper functioning. It includes not just the amount of food ingested, but also the quality and diversity of nutrients that the body requires. Balanced eating promotes general health, increases energy levels, and, most importantly, helps to maintain a healthy weight.

8.1.2 Mind-Body Connection in Nutrition:

I. Mindful Eating Practices:

1. Sensory Awareness: Somatics promotes increased sensory awareness, a concept that is effortlessly integrated with mindful eating practices. Engaging the senses when eating builds a stronger connection with the meal, which promotes appreciation and enjoyment.

2. Eating with Intention: Mindful eating is consistent with somatic intentionality. Instead of eating on autopilot, people are urged to approach meals with mindfulness, concentrating on the nutrients and pleasure of each mouthful.

8.1.3 Somatic Methods for Nutrient Absorption:

I. Breathwork and Digestion:

1. Diaphragmatic Breathing: Somatic techniques often include diaphragmatic breathing, which not only helps relaxation but also improves digestion. Individuals may optimize nutrition absorption by activating the diaphragm, which supports the digestive organs' natural rhythmic movement.

2. Stress Reduction: Chronic stress has a deleterious influence on digestion and nutrition absorption. Somatic techniques, with their stress-reduction advantages, help to create a more conducive environment for nutritional digestion.

8.1.4 Nutrition as Fuel for Somatic Movement:

I. Preparing Your Body for Exercise:

1. Balanced Macronutrients: An adequate diet guarantees that there is enough energy for somatic activity. The ratio of macronutrients—carbohydrates, proteins, and fats—is critical in delivering sustained energy for physical activity.

2. Hydration: Staying hydrated is essential for both somatic activities and general well-being. Hydrated muscles are more supple and receptive, allowing for smooth movement during somatic exercises.

8.1.5 Somatic Movement for Improved Metabolism:

I. Activating the Body's Natural Processes:

1. Gentle Cardiovascular Benefits: Somatic motions provide gentle cardiovascular exercise by improving circulation and maintaining a healthy metabolism. While somatic workouts are less strenuous than regular cardio, their rhythmic and purposeful nature stimulates the cardiovascular system.

2. Muscle Activation: A healthy metabolism relies heavily on the development and maintenance of lean muscle mass. Somatic exercises, which target multiple muscle groups, stimulate muscular activation without putting too much load on the body.

8.1.6 Personalizing Nutrition for Somatic Practices:

I. Meeting Individual Energy Needs:

1. Caloric Intake: People who engage in somatic activities may have different energy requirements. Nutrition must be tailored to these demands, taking into account aspects such as the intensity and length of somatic workouts.

2. Meal Timing: It is critical to align meal times with somatic activities. Consuming a balanced lunch or snack including carbs and protein before to indulging in somatic activities gives an appropriate energy supply.

8.1.7 Mind-Body Techniques for Emotional Eating:

I. Breaking the Cycle:

1. Body Awareness for Emotional Triggers: Somatic activities increase body awareness, allowing people to notice physical sensations linked to emotions. This increased awareness helps to disrupt the pattern of emotional eating by offering alternate coping techniques.

2. Mindful Food Choices: Incorporating somatic concepts with nutrition necessitates mindful food choices. This involves thinking about how food makes the body feel and selecting healthy alternatives that support somatic well-being.

8.1.8 Holistic Approaches to Weight Management:

I. Beyond Calorie Restriction:

1. Embracing Nourishment: Holistic weight control is more than just calorie restriction. It entails providing the body with nutritious, nutrient-dense meals that promote general well-being—a premise shared by somatics and nutrition.

2. ***Pleasant Relationship with Food:*** Somatic practices help to promote a pleasant relationship with food. Individuals who approach nutrition with mindfulness and purpose may overcome restricted diet mentalities and build a sustainable and balanced way of eating.

8.1.9 Addressing Individual Needs:

I. Customized Strategies for Success:

1. ***Body-Mind Variability:*** It is important to recognize that everyone has their distinct body-mind variances. Customizing both somatic practices and dietary techniques ensures that they meet an individual's unique requirements, preferences, and objectives.

2. *Flexibility in Approaches:* Somatics and nutrition both demand flexibility. Being willing to change strategies depending on individual reactions and changing circumstances adds to long-term success in comprehensive weight control.

The synergies between somatics and nutrition give a comprehensive approach to holistic weight control, taking into account the delicate relationship between mind and body. By incorporating somatic concepts into diet and vice versa, people go on a transformational journey that goes beyond traditional weight control measures. Holistic well-being is reached not via individual efforts, but through the harmonious integration of disciplines that feed both the body and the mind.

8.2 How to Improve the Impact of Somatic Practices with Mindful Eating

The combination of somatic activities with mindful eating forms a synergistic alliance that transcends standard health methods. Somatic activities, which emphasize the mind-body connection and deliberate movement, complement mindful eating—a strategy that promotes awareness, presence, and a deep connection with the process of feeding the body. Let dig into the complexities of maximizing the influence of somatic practices via mindful food choices, examining how this synergy leads to overall well-being and transformational personal development.

8.2.1 Understanding the Essence of Somatics Practices:

I. The Mind-Body Connection:

Somatic practices are based on the underlying idea of the mind-body connection. Unlike traditional workout regimens, somatics focuses on the interior sensation of movement, stressing awareness, intention, and the release of excess tension. Individuals go on a voyage of self-discovery via gentle exercises, breathwork, and increased body awareness, resulting in a better knowledge of their physical and mental condition.

II. Intentional Movement and Fluidity:

Somatic activities promote deliberate movement, with each action handled with a feeling of purpose and awareness. This systematic approach enables people to investigate the intricacies of their bodies' reactions, developing fluidity and flexibility in their motions. Somatic activities become a means of self-expression and self-care, allowing people to create a healthy connection with their bodies.

8.2.2 The Art of Mindful Eating:

I. Beyond Satiety:

Mindful eating applies the ideas of mindfulness and intention to the field of sustenance. It entails paying full attention throughout meals, relishing each mouthful, and developing a profound appreciation for the tastes, textures, and sustenance offered by the food. Mindful eating is more than just absorbing calories; it is a mindful and enjoyable experience of feeding the body.

II. The Mind-Body Dialogue:

1. Tuning into Hunger and Fullness: Mindful eating encourages people to pay attention to their bodies' signals of hunger and fullness. Through this heightened awareness, people learn to discriminate between bodily hunger and emotional needs, creating a more intuitive approach to feeding.

2. Sensory Exploration: Somatic practices and mindful eating both rely heavily on sensory engagement. Food textures, scents, and tastes become a sensory investigation, resulting in a harmonic interaction between the body and the sustenance it consumes.

8.2.3 Bridging Somatic Practices and Mindful Eating:

I. Developing a Unified Mind-Body Experience:

1. Pre-Meal Centering: Before meals, use somatic activities to center and ground oneself. To return your consciousness to the present moment, use mild motions, breathwork, or a quick body scan. This creates the conditions for a thoughtful and focused eating experience.

2. Mindful Bites: Treat each mouthful with the same thoughtfulness as somatic motions. Consciously chew and appreciate the tastes, making dining a thoughtful, embodied experience. This combination of somatics and mindful eating improves the total effect on the body and mind.

8.2.4 The Emotional Landscape Of Eating:

I. Navigating Emotional Eating Patterns:

1. Mindful Emotional Awareness: Somatic activities help people develop emotional awareness by helping them to examine and release tension. When applied to eating, this awareness enables people to notice emotional triggers and build mindful reactions to emotional signals rather than resorting to food for solace.

2. Embracing Emotional Resilience: Mindful eating, when paired with somatic activities, promotes emotional resilience. The capacity to traverse emotional landscapes without using food as a coping technique becomes an essential component of overall well-being.

8.2.5 Mindful Eating for Sustainable Weight Management:

I. Developing a Healthy Relationship with Food:

1. Breaking Free from Restrictive Diet Mentalities: Somatic techniques challenge stiff and forceful motions, encouraging ease and fluidity. Applying this idea to nutrition entails abandoning restricted diet mindsets. Mindful eating promotes a balanced and sustainable attitude to food, liberating people from the confines of strict dietary guidelines.

2. Cultivating Healthy Food Connections: Somatics and mindful eating both promote the development of healthy connections with movement and food. Individuals who approach meals with appreciation, curiosity, and a nonjudgmental attitude have a wholesome connection with the food they eat.

8.2.6 Somatic Practice and Digestive Harmony :

I. Facilitating Optimal Digestion:

1. Breathwork for Digestive Support: To aid digestion, use somatic breathwork methods. Diaphragmatic breathing, for example, promotes relaxation and may be especially effective before and after meals, helping to ensure proper digestive function.

2. Post-Meal Body Scan: After meals, do a quick body scan. This somatic technique helps to discover stress points and promotes the body's natural digestion functions. Individuals who maintain a calm state enhance effective digestion and nutrition absorption.

8.2.7 Mindful Food Choices for Somatic Nourishment:

I. Nutrient-Dense Selections:

1. Whole, Unprocessed Foods: Select whole, unprocessed foods that follow the principles of somatic well-being. These nutrient-dense, additive-free meals help the body operate optimally.

2. Hydration Practices: Build mindful drinking habits into your somatic journey. Drink water with focus, and think about herbal teas to help you relax. Proper hydration enhances both somatic practices and general health.

Individuals find a harmonic combination between somatic activities and mindful eating that goes beyond the limitations of standard health techniques. This synergy promotes not just physical well-being, but also a greater connection to oneself and the transforming power of mindful living.

CHAPTER 9: OVERCOMING OBSTACLES FOR LONG-TERM SUCCESS

9.1 Identifying and Addressing Common Obstacles in Somatic Exercise for Weight Control

Starting a somatic exercise journey for weight loss is a transforming experience that focuses on your whole well-being. However, like any worthwhile endeavor, it is not without its difficulties. This chapter looks into the identification and proactive resolution of major hurdles that people may face when including somatic exercise in their weight control routines. Individuals may manage their somatic journey with resilience by recognizing these problems and giving techniques for overcoming them, maintaining a long-term and good connection with their bodies.

9.1.1 Recognizing Common Obstacles to Somatic Exercise:

1. Perceived Lack of Intensity:

Challenge: Somatic exercises often favor soft, purposeful movements over high-intensity workouts. Some people may interpret this as a lack of efficacy, particularly if they are used to more strenuous workout regimens.

Addressing the Challenge:

1. Focus on the depth of somatic motions: Somatic exercises have a dramatic effect on the neurological system, alleviating stress and boosting general well-being.
2. Encourage consistency: Remind them that the cumulative effect of frequent somatic

practice is considerable, even if individual sessions may not seem intense.

2. Impatience with Results:

Challenge: In a society used to rapid cures, people may feel frustrated if a somatic activity does not provide instant weight reduction benefits.

Addressing the Challenge:

1. Prioritize holistic well-being: Change the emphasis from weight reduction to total well-being. Highlight the mental and emotional benefits of somatic exercise, emphasizing that sustainable weight management is a gradual process.

2. Create reasonable expectations: Encourage people to see their somatic journey as a long-term investment in health, with weight control being only one component of the bigger picture.

3. Resistance to Mindfulness Practices:

Challenge: Some people may struggle to accept the mindfulness part of somatic exercises, feeling resistive to techniques that require self-awareness and mental presence.

Addressing the Challenge:

1. Highlighting Mental Health Benefits: Emphasize that somatic techniques not only improve physical well-being but also offer significant mental health benefits. Increased self-awareness and stress reduction are key components of the practice.

2. Begin with Little Steps: Introduce mindfulness gradually, maybe by including small periods of awareness throughout sessions. Encourage people to explore at their speed.

4. Time Constraints:

Challenge: Consistent somatic practice might be challenging due to busy lives and schedules.

Addressing the Challenge:

1. Focus on short, effective sessions: Emphasize that somatic exercises may be incorporated into everyday routines via brief, powerful sessions. It is not necessarily about the time, but rather the consistency of practice.

2. Encourage time management: Assist folks in identifying time pockets for somatic practice in their daily lives. Emphasize that even small periods of focused movement add to the total benefits.

5. Need for External Validation:

Challenge: Relying on external validation, such as physical changes or cultural standards, may be challenging for those who do not get instant recognition for their efforts.

Addressing the Challenge:

Foster internal validation: Encourage internal validation by recognizing and celebrating internal improvements like better posture, lower tension, and enhanced bodily awareness. Remind them that somatic exercise is a personal journey, and external validation may not necessarily reflect individual improvement.

6. Fear of Judgment:

Challenge: Fear of judgment, whether from others or self-judgment, might prevent persons from completely participating in somatic activities.

Addressing the Challenge:

1. Create a supportive atmosphere and emphasize the non-judgmental character of somatic activities. Create a feeling of

community and support inside group sessions by providing a secure environment for people to explore and express themselves.

2. Promote self-compassion: Remind people that somatic exercise is a personal journey with no need for self-judgment. Encourage self-compassion and a focus on the journey rather than the apparent outcome.

9.1.2 Strategies to Overcome Common Obstacles

1. Education and Communication:

Strategy: Provide in-depth information on the concepts and advantages of somatic exercises. Establish lines of communication to resolve issues and misinformation.

2. Goal-setting and Progress Tracking:

Strategy: Facilitate goal-setting sessions that concentrate on overall health rather than just weight reduction. Encourage people to keep track of their development, acknowledging both apparent and internal improvements.

3. Gradual Integration of Mindfulness:

Strategy: Gradually integrate mindfulness techniques into somatic sessions, allowing people to relax into the mental parts of the practice at their speed.

4. Flexible Practice Options:

Strategy: Provide a wide range of somatic workouts that may be tailored to varied time limitations. Allow for session duration flexibility and encourage people to adjust their practice to their schedules.

5. Mindfulness Training Workshops:

Strategy: Hold mindfulness-focused seminars to assist people in understanding its advantages and provide practical techniques for implementing it into their everyday lives.

6. Encourage Peer Support:

Strategy: Create a feeling of community in somatic exercise groups to share experiences, encourage one another, and reduce fear of criticism.

7. Body Positivity and Self-Love Workshops:

Strategy: Hold seminars encouraging body acceptance and self-love. Encourage people to accept their bodies as they are and to appreciate the importance of somatic activities beyond looks.

Identifying and resolving frequent difficulties in somatic exercise for weight control is an important part of empowering people on their transformational path. Practitioners and educators play an important role in building a resilient and good connection between people and their somatic practices by raising awareness of possible problems and giving techniques for overcoming them.

9.2 Creating Strategies for Long-Term Adherence to Somatic Exercise for Weight Management

Starting a somatic exercise journey for weight loss is more than simply setting short-term objectives; it's a commitment to a lifestyle that values overall well-being. Sustained, long-term dedication is the key to success in this revolutionary undertaking. This chapter delves into the creation of ways to create a long-term commitment to somatic exercise, ensuring that people not only meet their weight management objectives but also effortlessly incorporate somatic practices into their daily lives for long-term health and vitality.

9.2.1 Understanding The Dynamics of Long-Term Commitment:

1. Holistic Goal Setting:

Foundational Aspect: Clarity and resonance of objectives are essential for long-term commitment.

Change the emphasis from weight-related goals to overall well-being. Emphasize that greater mobility, lower stress, and improved general health are all worthwhile results.

2. Intrinsic Motivation:

Motivational Factor: Intrinsic motivation drives long-term commitment. Assist people in identifying their motivations for participating in somatic exercise, such as a desire for more energy, stress relief, or enhanced mental clarity. Intrinsic motives typically motivate long-term commitment more efficiently than extrinsic reasons.

3. Progress Tracking:

Monitoring Tool: Set up a method for monitoring progress. Re-evaluate objectives regularly, recognize accomplishments, and adjust techniques to meet changing requirements. Tracking progress gives a concrete indication of the good influence that somatic exercise has on one's well-being, instilling a feeling of success.

4. Consistency Over Intensity:

Mindset Shift: Encourage a mentality change from chasing hard, infrequent exercises to consistent, focused movements. Point out that the cumulative impact of frequent, mild somatic exercises outweighs the advantages of occasional, hard workouts. Consistency creates the foundation for long-term commitment.

5. Developing Mindfulness Habits:

Lifestyle Integration: Incorporate mindfulness practices into your everyday life. Encourage people to integrate somatic concepts into their everyday activities, such as sitting with good posture, breathing intentionally while working, and taking brief movement breaks. This seamless connection promotes a lifestyle in which somatic actions are second nature.

9.2.2 Strategies for Maintaining Long-Term Commitment:

1. Holistic Well Being Workshops:
Educational Initiative: Hold seminars that explore the overall advantages of somatic exercise. Examine how it improves mental wellness, stress reduction, and general vitality. Fostering complete knowledge promotes the commitment to a healthy lifestyle.

2. Individualized Practice Plan:
Tailored Approach: Work together to create specific somatic practice programs. Recognize the individuality of each individual's physique and preferences. A personalized approach ensures that the practice fits with their lifestyle, making long-term commitment more attainable.

3. Mind-Body Check-Ins:
Regular Reflection: Establish regular mind-body check-ins so people may reflect on their somatic

journey. These check-ins allow participants to analyze how the practice affects their general well-being, developing a stronger connection and dedication to the transformational process.

4. Community Engagement:

Support Network: Create a feeling of community for those on the somatic journey. Create forums for exchanging experiences, difficulties, and successes. A supportive community offers encouragement in times of uncertainty, strengthening the commitment to continuous somatic activities.

5. Integrative Lifestyle Sessions:

Practical Application: Organize workshops to show how somatic concepts may be smoothly incorporated into everyday life. Investigate methods to combine deliberate movements, breathwork, and mindfulness into a variety of tasks. Making somatic practices more practical and useful increases their sustainability.

6. Mindfulness Rituals:

Daily Integration: Encourage the creation of everyday thoughtful practices. This might include a morning breathwork routine, a lunchtime mobility break, or an evening relaxing session. Establishing these rituals provides a regular context for somatic activities, reaffirming their importance in everyday life.

7. Personalized Reinforcement Techniques:

Positive Reinforcement: Work with people to develop tailored reinforcement strategies. This might include setting reminders, producing visual signals, or constructing a reward system based on persistent somatic practice. Personalized reinforcement strategies improve the commitment loop.

8. Seasonal Adaptations:

Flexible Approach: Recognize that different obstacles may arise at different stages of life. Create techniques for adjusting somatic activities to changing seasons, such as hectic job times, family responsibilities, or personal issues. A flexible attitude allows for life's fluctuations.

9. Education about Long-Term Benefits:

Informative Approach: Continuously educate people about the long-term advantages of somatic exercise. Provide insights on how these behaviors help to maintain health, energy, and resilience. A thorough grasp of the long-term consequences encourages dedication beyond current aims.

10. Celebrating Milestones:

Recognition Ritual: Establish a culture of recognizing accomplishments, both large and small. Recognize gains in mobility, stress reduction, and general well-being. Celebrations foster pleasant connections with somatic activities, emphasizing their importance.

Sustained, long-term dedication to somatic exercise for weight control is a never-ending path toward lifetime well-being. By using these tactics, practitioners and people alike may cultivate a commitment that goes beyond transient aims, adopting a lifestyle in which somatic activities become an intrinsic and lasting component of everyday living. May the path be one of self-discovery, resilience, and deep connection—a dedication that goes beyond the physical to include the very essence of well-being.

CHAPTER 10: SOMATICS BEYOND WEIGHT

10.1 Investigating the Broader Benefits of Somatics Practices for Overall Well-Being

Somatic practices, which are often connected with particular movement modalities and mindfulness approaches, extend far beyond their apparent limitations. While first recognized for their influence on physical health and weight control, these practices have far-reaching consequences for complete well-being, including mental, emotional, and spiritual aspects. This chapter delves into the wide range of benefits that somatic practices provide, offering light on how they contribute to a holistic and transforming path toward overall well-being.

10.1.1 A Holistic Approach to Well-Being:

1. Physical Vitality:

I. ***Muscular Release and Tension Reduction:*** Feldenkrais and BodyMind Centering are examples of somatic techniques that emphasize the release of muscular tension. Individuals develop a greater awareness of their bodies via gentle and focused movements, which allows for muscle release and increased overall physical vigor.

II. ***Improved Flexibility and Range of Motion:*** Somatic exercises aim to release restrictive movement patterns, resulting in increased flexibility and a wider range of motion. This not only helps to increase physical performance but also lowers the risk of injuries caused by stiffness and restricted movement.

2. Mental Clarity:

I. ***Nervous System Regulation:*** Somatic techniques actively work with the nervous system to promote regulation and balance. Mindful movement and breathwork help to soothe the nervous system, reduce tension, and improve mental clarity. People often report enhanced attention, concentration, and cognitive performance as a consequence.

II. ***Mind-Body Connection:*** The focus on the mind-body link in somatic practices promotes a greater understanding of how mental states affect physical well-being. This increased connection enables people to face everyday obstacles with more resilience and mental clarity.

3. Emotional Resilience:

I. ***Release of Emotional Tension:*** Somatic techniques provide a safe environment for the release of emotional tension held in the body. Individuals may explore and release emotions using mindful movements and breathwork, which promotes emotional resilience and well-being.

II. ***Mindful Processing of Emotions:*** The attentive nature of somatic activities allows people to analyze and comprehend their feelings in real-time. This increased emotional awareness helps emotional intelligence, enabling more deliberate reactions to life's ups and downs.

4. Stress Reduction:

I. ***Breathwork Methods:*** Many somatic disciplines use specialized breathwork methods to influence the body's stress response. Diaphragmatic breathing and other deliberate breath activities stimulate the parasympathetic nervous system, resulting in relaxation and stress reduction.

II. **_Tension Pattern Release:_** Muscular tension patterns are a common manifestation of chronic stress. Somatic exercises, with their gentle and exploratory character, assist people in identifying and releasing tension patterns, fostering a long-term sensation of calm and resistance to stress.

5. Spiritual Connection:

I. **_Embodied Presence:_** Somatic practices stress embodied presence, which is the act of completely experiencing one's body in the present time. This emphasis on presence promotes a feeling of spiritual connection, enabling people to delve into their inner selves and build a deep connection to the world around them.

II. *Mindful Awareness:* The mindfulness inherent in somatic techniques goes beyond the physical domain to include a larger understanding of life's interdependence. This increased awareness may lead to a feeling of spiritual satisfaction and purpose.

10.1.2 The Transformational Power of Somatic Practices

1. Enhanced Body Awareness:

I. *Mindful Movement:* Somatic activities promote mindful movement, helping people to become aware of their bodies' subtle signals and feelings. This increased bodily awareness lasts beyond the exercise session, encouraging a constant level of mindfulness in everyday life.

II. *Prevention of Overuse Injuries*: Increased bodily awareness allows people to detect early indicators of tension or strain, lowering their risk of overuse injuries. This preventative element helps to maintain bodily well-being.

2. Improved Posture and Alignment:

I. ***Reeducation of Movement Patterns***: Somatic techniques retrain movement patterns, correcting postural abnormalities and encouraging healthy alignment. Improved posture not only benefits physical health but also affects how people carry themselves, instilling confidence and well-being.

II. ***Chronic Pain Reduction:*** Poor posture and movement patterns are common causes of chronic pain. Somatic exercises, which target the underlying causes of pain, help to reduce or eliminate chronic pain, improving general comfort and well-being.

3. Emotional Regulation:

I. ***Balancing Emotional States:*** Somatic techniques provide strategies for achieving emotional balance. Individuals may transition from anxious or agitated situations to tranquility and emotional balance by using focused movements and breathwork.

II. ***Integration of Mind and Emotion:*** The mind-body link inherent in somatic activities enables the integration of mind and emotion. This integration promotes emotional harmony, resulting in a more balanced and robust emotional environment.

4. Mindful Living:

I. ***Daily Mindfulness Integration:*** Somatic activities facilitate the incorporation of mindfulness into one's everyday life. Whether sitting at a computer, strolling, or engaged in ordinary tasks, people learn to apply deliberate awareness to their motions, promoting a continual state of mindful life.

II. ***Tension Prevention:*** By bringing mindfulness into regular activities, people may avoid building up tension throughout the day. This proactive approach to stress avoidance promotes long-term well-being and a more balanced lifestyle.

10.1.3 Promoting Overall Well-Being Through Somatic Practices

1. Holistic Self-Care Practices:

I. ***Nourishing the Whole Self:*** Somatic activities evolve into a sort of comprehensive self-care that addresses the individual's physical, mental, emotional, and spiritual needs. This holistic method nurtures the whole person, generating a feeling of wholeness and well-being.

II. *Self-Love Cultivation:* Somatic techniques promote self-love and acceptance. Individuals learn to enjoy and care for themselves via focused movements and a nonjudgmental examination of the body.

2. Empowerment and Autonomy:

I. *Embodied Empowerment:* Somatic techniques empower people by instilling a feeling of control over their health. The capacity to relieve stress, control emotions, and boost physical vigor fosters a sense of autonomy and empowerment.

II. *Self-Directed Well-Being:* Somatic practices provide people with the skills they need to manage their well-being. Individuals who practice self-awareness and mindfulness may actively engage in their path to general health and satisfaction.

As people discover the greater benefits of somatic practices, they go on a transforming journey that goes well beyond physical health. Somatic activities serve as a doorway to general well-being, weaving together threads of physical vitality, mental clarity, emotional resilience, and spiritual connection. Within this comprehensive framework, the full nature and transformational potential of somatic activities emerge. As the journey progresses, may the comprehensive essence of somatic practices continue to reveal the route to a life profoundly enhanced by the transformational power of aware, deliberate living.

10.2 Adopting Sustainable Health Practices for a Fulfilling and Balanced Lifestyle

Adopting sustainable health habits is critical in the pursuit of a full and balanced life. Beyond fads and fast cures, sustainable health practices provide the groundwork for long-term well-being, guiding people through the difficulties of contemporary life while maintaining their physical, mental, and emotional vigor. This chapter delves into the essential ideas and tactics for building long-term health behaviors that lead to a fulfilling and balanced lifestyle.

10.2.1 Understanding Sustainable Healthcare Practices:

1. Holistic Wellbeing:

Integration of Physical, Mental, and Emotional Health: Sustainable health practices use a comprehensive approach that considers physical, mental, and emotional well-being. Recognizing the connection of these components is critical to living a balanced and fulfilled life.

Long-Term Focus: Unlike quick solutions, sustainable health approaches promote long-term results. This entails building habits and routines that lead to long-term vitality rather than pursuing instant outcomes that may not be sustained over time.

2. Mindful Living:

Present-Moment Awareness: Mindful living is the foundation of sustainable health practices. It entails growing present-moment awareness in everyday tasks, as well as taking a deliberate and purposeful approach to eating, activity, and general lifestyle choices.

Connection to Somatic Practices: Somatic practices, which emphasize attentive movement and breathwork, are perfectly aligned with the ideals of mindful living. Incorporating somatic exercises into everyday activities helps to integrate awareness into many facets of life.

10.2.2 Key Principles for Sustainable Healthcare Practices

1. Personalisation and Flexibility:
Tailoring Practices to Individual Requirements: Recognizing that each person is unique, sustainable health practices need methods that are tailored to individual requirements and preferences. This may include tailoring exercise regimens, food choices, and self-care practices to match personal objectives and lifestyles.

Adaptability to Life Changes: Sustainable health practices are flexible enough to adjust to life's variations. Whether dealing with hectic work schedules, family obligations, or unexpected problems, the capacity to adapt to changing circumstances ensures that health habits remain consistent throughout life.

2. Developing Positive Habits:

Progressive Implementation: Sustainable health practices are based on progressive habit building. Rather than making dramatic adjustments, people are urged to adopt new habits gradually, allowing for a more lasting incorporation into everyday life.

Emphasize Consistency: The focus is on tiny, consistent acts that add up over time. Individuals may create the framework for long-term health gains by concentrating on developing beneficial habits daily, rather than forcing sudden changes.

3. Accepting Diversity in Movement and Nutrition:

Incorporating Diverse Exercise Modalities: Adopting various types of activity is essential for a long-term approach to physical wellness. This might include a mix of aerobic workouts, weight training, and somatic techniques to address various elements of fitness and avoid boredom.

Balanced and Pleasurable Nutrition: Sustainable nutrition practices emphasize a well-balanced and pleasurable eating experience. Rather than rigorous diets, people are urged to have a healthy connection with food, including a range of nutrient-dense selections while enjoying the delights of eating.

4. Mindful Stress Management:

Holistic Stress Reduction Techniques: Sustainable health practices put a high value on holistic stress reduction. Meditation, breathwork, and somatic exercises are helpful strategies for stress management, resilience building, and burnout prevention.

Rest and Recovery Integration: Sustainable health practices emphasize the significance of rest and recovery by promoting appropriate sleep, downtime, and relaxation. These components are essential for sustaining general well-being and avoiding the detrimental consequences of prolonged stress.

5. Community and Support Networks:

Creating a Supportive Community: A supportive community encourages long-term health behaviors. A community, whether in the form of fitness groups, nutrition forums, or mindfulness circles, promotes encouragement, shared experiences, and mutual support.

Social Connections and Mental Health: Recognizing the importance of social connections for mental health, sustainable practices focus on sustaining relationships and cultivating a feeling of belonging.

Strong social bonds promote emotional well-being and resilience.

10.2.3 Strategies for Adopting Sustainable Healthcare Practices:

1. Education and Empowerment:

Informed Decision-Making: Education and empowerment are key strategies for implementing sustainable health practices. Individuals are encouraged to make educated health decisions by knowing the underlying concepts, whether they are connected to diet, exercise, or stress management.

Cultivating a Growth Mentality: Having a growth mentality is essential. Embracing difficulties, perceiving failures as learning opportunities, and knowing that health is a dynamic journey all help to foster a sustainable mentality.

2. Setting Goals and Keeping Track of Progress:

Setting Realistic and Personalized Goals: Setting realistic, individualized objectives that are consistent with an individual's beliefs and ambitions is a key component of sustainable health practice. These objectives act as progress indicators and give guidance on the path to well-being.

Regular Progress Monitoring: Individuals are encouraged to keep track of their progress, celebrate accomplishments, and change objectives as appropriate. This continual examination promotes self-awareness and ensures that health approaches stay relevant to changing demands.

3. Integrating Somatic Practices:

Increasing Mindfulness and Body Awareness: Integrating somatic activities like mindful movement and breathwork improves mindfulness and body awareness. These techniques become effective tools for connecting with the body and developing a better knowledge of its signals and demands.

Tension Reduction and Emotional Regulation: Somatic techniques help to relieve tension and regulate emotions. Individuals who include these tactics in their daily routines improve their ability to handle stress and create emotional resilience, both of which are essential components of long-term health.

4. Developing a Positive Mindset:

Positive Self-talk and Self-Compassion: Adopting sustainable health habits necessitates developing a good attitude. Individuals are urged to use positive self-talk, exercise self-compassion, and face problems with resilience. A positive mentality encourages the continuation of health activities throughout different living conditions.

Appreciation for Progress: Recognizing and praising progress, no matter how tiny, promotes a good attitude. Recognizing accomplishments, reinforcing motivation, and cultivating a feeling of contentment on the path to well-being are all components of sustainable health practices.

Adopting sustainable health habits is a continuous journey toward satisfaction and balance. When people embrace the ideas of holistic well-being, mindful living, and various health techniques, they pave the path for a life full of energy, resilience, and satisfaction. May this chapter serve as a compass, guiding people toward habits that not only improve their physical health but also add to the rich tapestry of a balanced and fulfilled existence.

CONCLUSION

As we come to the end of our voyage into the transformational world of somatic exercise for weight loss and general well-being, we reflect on the rich tapestry that has been created throughout. From the fundamental principles of somatic practices to the subtle integration of mindfulness into everyday life, the chapters of this book have served as a guide—an invitation to begin on a comprehensive path toward long-term well-being.

Reflecting on Key Themes

1. Somatic Exercise as a Paradigm Shift: The journey started with a transition from conventional fitness practices to somatic exercise. This transformation included seeing the body as a dynamic, linked system in which movement is more than just a physical activity but also a doorway to improved body awareness, stress management, and emotional resilience.

2. *Mind-Body Connection is the Anchor:* Somatic exercise relies heavily on the mind-body connection. Chapters explored the complex relationship between the neurological system, stress hormones, and the skill of restoring inner knowledge. This link became the guiding thread, allowing people to negotiate the intricacies of weight control with awareness and purpose.

3. *Embracing Holistic Health And Dispelling Myths:* The voyage debunked many misconceptions about weight reduction, questioning traditional calorie calculations and easy fixes. Instead, it argued for a more holistic approach, seeing weight control as simply one aspect of total well-being. This holistic viewpoint encouraged people to go beyond cultural classifications and discover the underlying advantages of somatic activities for a fulfilled existence.

4. Somatic Practices as Personalized Transformation:
The chapters provide a roadmap for individualized
change, highlighting the significance of specific
somatic workout routines. Individuals were
encouraged to develop practices that were tailored
to their requirements, interests, and lifestyles,
ranging from embodied movement and breathwork
to mindful eating.

5. Additional Benefits Beyond Weight Loss: The
research went beyond weight reduction to reveal
the wider advantages of somatic activities for
overall health. It demonstrated how somatic
exercises promote physical health, mental clarity,
emotional resilience, and even spiritual
connectedness. Somatic practices evolved as
catalysts for a comprehensive change that extends
beyond the physical sphere.

6. Navigating Challenges with Resilience: This theme
emphasizes the importance of overcoming barriers

on the way to long-term well-being. Whether tackling common challenges, building long-term commitment methods, or investigating the synergy between somatics and nutrition, the trip emphasized perseverance in the face of hardship.

7. *Integration into Daily Life:* The trip demonstrated that lasting well-being extends beyond exercise sessions and pervades all aspects of life. From mindful movement to conscious food choices, people were enabled to build a lifestyle in which somatic practices were ingrained in their being.

The Power of Somatic Practices Unveiled:

As we close, the transforming potential of somatic practices is revealed—power that goes beyond physical fitness and beyond the traditional confines of exercise. Somatic practices evolve into a philosophy—a way of life that cultivates awareness strengthens the mind-body connection, and promotes resilience in the face of life's challenges.

This journey is not limited to the pages of this book; it encompasses people's everyday decisions, deliberate moves, and attentive moments. It is a journey that takes place in quiet areas of self-reflection, decisions made at the dinner table, and intentional moments of connection with the body's intrinsic knowledge.

A Lifetime Commitment to Holistic Well-Being:
As readers complete the chapters of this book, we encourage them to take the spirit of somatic practices forward—a dedication to holistic well-being that goes beyond weight reduction and pervades every aspect of life. The trip continues, not as a destination, but as a lifetime exploration—a tapestry of deliberate decisions, conscious moves, and changing experiences. Individuals should embrace the resilience developed via somatic activities, appreciate achievements, and handle adversities with grace.

Finally, May they find satisfaction in the developing path toward long-term well-being—a journey that goes far beyond the physical to include the whole essence of life. Let the principles of somatic exercise serve as a compass, directing people toward a life of vitality, awareness, and long-term well-being.

NOTE

<u>NOTE</u>